ORTHOPEDIC CLINICS OF NORTH AMERICA

www.orthopedic.theclinics.com

Outpatient Surgery

January 2018 • Volume 49 • Number 1

ELSEVIER

1600 John F. Kennedy Boulevard • Suite 1800 • Philadelphia, Pennsylvania, 19103-2899.

http://www.orthopedic.theclinics.com

ORTHOPEDIC CLINICS OF NORTH AMERICA Volume 49, Number 1
January 2018 ISSN 0030-5898, ISBN-13: 978-0-323-56645-2

Editor: Lauren Boyle
Developmental Editor: Kristen Helm

Orthopedic Clinics of North America (ISSN 0030-5898) is published quarterly by Elsevier Inc., 360 Park Avenue South, New York, NY 10010-1710. Months of issue are January, April, July, and October. Business and Editorial Offices: 1600 John F. Kennedy Blvd., Suite 1800, Philadelphia, PA 19103-2899. Customer Service Office: 3251 Riverport Lane, Maryland Heights, MO 63043. Periodicals postage paid at New York, NY and additional mailing offices. Subscription prices are $332.00 per year for (US individuals), $713.00 per year for (US institutions), $391.00 per year (Canadian individuals), $870.00 per year (Canadian institutions), $464.00 per year (international individuals), $870.00 per year (international institutions), $100.00 per year (US students), $220.00 per year (Canadian and international students). Foreign air speed delivery is included in all *Clinics* subscription prices. All prices are subject to change without notice. **POSTMASTER:** Send change of address to *Orthopedic Clinics of North America,* **Elsevier Health Sciences Division, Subscription Customer Service, 3251 Riverport Lane, Maryland Heights, MO 63043. Customer Service (orders, claims, online, change of address):** Elsevier Health Sciences Division, Subscription Customer Service, 3251 Riverport Lane, Maryland Heights, MO 63043. Tel: **1-800-654-2452 (U.S. and Canada); 314-447-8871 (outside U.S. and Canada). Fax: 314-447-8029. E-mail:** journalscustomerservice-usa@elsevier.com **(for print support);** journalsonlinesupport-usa@elsevier.com **(for online support).**

Reprints. For copies of 100 or more, of articles in this publication, please contact the Commercial Reprints Department, Elsevier Inc., 360 Park Avenue South, New York, NY 10010-1710. Tel.: 212-633-3874; Fax: 212-633-3820; E-mail: reprints@elsevier.com.

Orthopedic Clinics of North America is covered in *MEDLINE/PubMed* (*Index Medicus*), *Cinahl, Excerpta Medica,* and *Cumulative Index to Nursing and Allied Health Literature.*

PROGRAM OBJECTIVE

Orthopedic Clinics of North America offers clinical review articles on the most cutting-edge technologies and techniques in the field, including adult reconstruction, the upper extremity, pediatrics, trauma, oncology, and sports medicine.

TARGET AUDIENCE

Practicing orthopedic surgeons, orthopedic residents, and other healthcare professionals who specialize in orthopedic technologies and techniques for adult reconstruction, the upper extremity, pediatrics, trauma, oncology, and sports medicine.

LEARNING OBJECTIVES

Upon completion of this activity, participants will be able to:
1. Review procedures and outcomes for outpatient total joint replacements.
2. Discuss outpatient surgeries for orthopedic traumas in pediatric and adult populations.
3. Recognize updates in procedures and pain management strategies for ambulatory surgeries of the extremities.

ACCREDITATION

The Elsevier Office of Continuing Medical Education (EOCME) is accredited by the Accreditation Council for Continuing Medical Education (ACCME) to provide continuing medical education for physicians.

The EOCME designates this enduring material for a maximum of 15 *AMA PRA Category 1 Credit*(s)™. Physicians should claim only the credit commensurate with the extent of their participation in the activity.

All other healthcare professionals requesting continuing education credit for this enduring material will be issued a certificate of participation.

DISCLOSURE OF CONFLICTS OF INTEREST

The EOCME assesses conflict of interest with its instructors, faculty, planners, and other individuals who are in a position to control the content of CME activities. All relevant conflicts of interest that are identified are thoroughly vetted by EOCME for fair balance, scientific objectivity, and patient care recommendations. EOCME is committed to providing its learners with CME activities that promote improvements or quality in healthcare and not a specific proprietary business or a commercial interest.

The planning committee, staff, authors and editors listed below have identified no financial relationships or relationships to products or devices they or their spouse/life partner have with commercial interest related to the content of this CME activity:

Leila Abaab, MD; Eric A. Barcak, DO; Nahum Michael Beard, MD, CAQSM; Michael J. Beebe, MD; Lauren Boyle; Tyler J. Brolin, MD; James H. Calandruccio, MD; Jason L. Codding, MD; Robert G. Dekker II, MD; Mouhanad El-Othmani, MD; John (Jack) M. Flynn, MD; Anjali Fortna; Wm. Grant Franco, BS; Theodore J. Ganley, MD; Charles L. Getz, MD; Robert Patrick Gousse, MD; Mia M. Helfrich, MD; Andrew Krause, MD; Leah Logan; Danielle Lovett-Carter, MD; William M. Mihalko, MD, PhD; Daniel J. Miller, MD; Susan E. Nelson, MD, MPH; Vinay Pallekonda, MD; Charles Qin, MD; Khaled J. Saleh, MD, MSc, FRCS(C), MHCM, CPE; Zain Sayeed, MD, MHA; Apurva S. Shah, MD, MBA; Murphy M. Steiner, MD; Jeyanthi Surendrakumar; Norfleet B. Thompson, MD.

The planning committee, staff, authors and editors listed below have identified financial relationships or relationships to products or devices they or their spouse/life partner have with commercial interest related to the content of this CME activity:

Anish R. Kadakia, MD receives royalties/patents from Acumed, A Colson Associate.
Paul Sethi, MD is on the speakers' bureau for, and is a consultant/advisor for, Arthrex, Inc; Pacira Pharmaceuticals; and Johnson & Johnson Services, Inc, has research support from Arthrex, Inc and Pacira Pharmaceuticals, and receives royalties/patents from Arthrex, Inc.
Thomas (Quin) Throckmorton, MD has stock ownership in Gilead, has research support from Zimmer Biomet, and receives royalties/patents from Zimmer Biomet.
John C. Weinlein, MD receives royalties from Elsevier.

UNAPPROVED/OFF-LABEL USE DISCLOSURE

The EOCME requires CME faculty to disclose to the participants:
1. When products or procedures being discussed are off-label, unlabelled, experimental, and/or investigational (not US Food and Drug Administration [FDA] approved); and
2. Any limitations on the information presented, such as data that are preliminary or that represent ongoing research, interim analyses, and/or unsupported opinions. Faculty may discuss information about pharmaceutical agents that is outside of FDA-approved labelling. This information is intended solely for CME and is not intended to promote off-label use of these medications. If you have any questions, contact the medical affairs department of the manufacturer for the most recent prescribing information.

TO ENROLL

To enroll in the *Orthopedic Clinics of North America* Continuing Medical Education program, call customer service at 1-800-654-2452 or sign up online at http://www.theclinics.com/home/cme. The CME program is available to subscribers for an additional annual fee of USD 215.

METHOD OF PARTICIPATION

In order to claim credit, participants must complete the following:

1. Complete enrolment as indicated above.
2. Read the activity.
3. Complete the CME Test and Evaluation. Participants must achieve a score of 70% on the test. All CME Tests and Evaluations must be completed online.

CME INQUIRIES/SPECIAL NEEDS

For all CME inquiries or special needs, please contact elsevierCME@elsevier.com.

EDITORIAL BOARD

BENJAMIN M. MAUCK, MD – HAND AND WRIST
Hand and Upper Extremity Surgery, Campbell Clinic; Clinical Instructor,
Department of Orthopedic Surgery, University of Tennessee Health Science
Center, Memphis, Tennessee

JAMES H. CALANDRUCCIO, MD – HAND AND WRIST
Assistant Professor, Department of Orthopaedic Surgery and Biomedical
Engineering, University of Tennessee-Campbell Clinic; Staff Physician, Campbell
Clinic, Inc, Memphis, Tennessee

THOMAS (QUIN) THROCKMORTON, MD – SHOULDER AND ELBOW
Professor, Shoulder and Elbow Surgery, Residency Program Director,
Department of Orthopaedic Surgery, University of Tennessee-Campbell Clinic,
Memphis Tennessee

CLAYTON C. BETTIN, MD – FOOT AND ANKLE
Instructor, Department of Orthopaedic Surgery and Biomedical Engineering,
University of Tennessee-Campbell Clinic; Staff Physician, Campbell Clinic, Inc,
Memphis, Tennessee

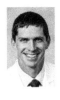

BENJAMIN J. GREAR, MD – FOOT AND ANKLE
Instructor, Department of Orthopaedic Surgery and Biomedical Engineering,
University of Tennessee-Campbell Clinic; Staff Physician, Campbell Clinic, Inc,
Memphis, Tennessee

CONTRIBUTORS

AUTHORS

LEILA ABAAB, MD
Departments of Orthopaedics and
Anesthesiology, NorthStar Anesthesia, Detroit
Medical Center, Detroit, Michigan

ERIC A. BARCAK, DO
Department of Orthopaedic
Surgery, University of Tennessee-Campbell
Clinic, Regional One Health, Memphis,
Tennessee

NAHUM MICHAEL BEARD, MD, CAQSM
Departments of Family Medicine
and Orthopedics and Rehabilitation,
Assistant Professor, The University of
Tennessee Health Science Center,
Memphis, Tennessee

MICHAEL J. BEEBE, MD
Department of Orthopaedic Surgery,
University of Tennessee-Campbell Clinic,
Regional One Health, Memphis, Tennessee

TYLER J. BROLIN, MD
Instructor, Shoulder and
Elbow Surgery, Department of
Orthopaedic Surgery, University of
Tennessee-Campbell Clinic, Memphis,
Tennessee

JAMES H. CALANDRUCCIO, MD
Associate Professor, Department
of Orthopaedic Surgery and
Biomedical Engineering, University of
Tennessee-Campbell Clinic, Memphis,
Tennessee

JASON L. CODDING, MD
Rothman Institute at Thomas
Jefferson University, Department of
Orthopaedic Surgery, Philadelphia,
Pennsylvania

ROBERT G. DEKKER II, MD
Department of Orthopedic
Surgery, Northwestern University,
Chicago, Illinois

MOUHANAD EL-OTHMANI, MD
Department of Orthopaedics, Detroit Medical
Center, Detroit, Michigan

JOHN (JACK) M. FLYNN, MD
Division of Orthopaedic Surgery, Children's
Hospital of Philadelphia, Philadelphia,
Pennsylvania

WM. GRANT FRANCO, BS
ONS Foundation for Clinical Research &
Education, Greenwich, Connecticut

THEODORE J. GANLEY, MD
Division of Orthopaedic Surgery, Children's
Hospital of Philadelphia, Philadelphia,
Pennsylvania

CHARLES L. GETZ, MD
Rothman Institute at Thomas
Jefferson University, Department of
Orthopaedic Surgery, Philadelphia,
Pennsylvania

ROBERT PATRICK GOUSSE, MD
Fellow, Primary Care Sports Medicine
Fellowship, Departments of Family Medicine
and Orthopedics and Rehabilitation, The
University of Tennessee Health Science
Center, Memphis, Tennessee

MIA M. HELFRICH, MD
Department of Orthopedic Surgery,
Northwestern University, Chicago, Illinois

ANISH R. KADAKIA, MD
Associate Professor of Orthopedic
Surgery, Foot and Ankle, Program
Director, Foot and Ankle Orthopedic
Fellowship, Department of Orthopedic
Surgery, Northwestern Memorial Hospital,
Northwestern University Feinberg School of
Medicine, Chicago, Illinois

ANDREW KRAUSE, MD
Department of Orthopaedics, Detroit Medical
Center, Detroit, Michigan

DANIELLE LOVETT-CARTER, MD
Department of Orthopaedics, Detroit Medical Center, Detroit, Michigan

WILLIAM M. MIHALKO, MD, PhD
Campbell Clinic Department of Orthopaedic Surgery & Biomedical Engineering University of Tennessee, Memphis, Tennessee

DANIEL J. MILLER, MD
Division of Orthopaedic Surgery, Children's Hospital of Philadelphia, Philadelphia, Pennsylvania

SUSAN E. NELSON, MD, MPH
Division of Orthopaedic Surgery, Children's Hospital of Philadelphia, Philadelphia, Pennsylvania

VINAY PALLEKONDA, MD
Department of Anesthesiology, NorthStar Anesthesia, Detroit Medical Center, Detroit, Michigan

CHARLES QIN, MD
Department of Orthopedic Surgery, The University of Chicago Medicine, Chicago, Illinois

KHALED J. SALEH, MD, MSc, FRCS(C), MHCM, CPE
Chairman, Department of Orthopaedics, Detroit Medical Center, Detroit, Michigan

ZAIN SAYEED, MD, MHA
Department of Orthopaedics, Detroit Medical Center, Detroit, Michigan

PAUL SETHI, MD
ONS Sports and Shoulder Service, President, ONS Foundation for Clinical Research and Education, Clinical Instructor in Orthopedic Surgery, Greenwich, Connecticut

APURVA S. SHAH, MD, MBA
Division of Orthopaedic Surgery, Children's Hospital of Philadelphia, Philadelphia, Pennsylvania

MURPHY M. STEINER, MD
Surgeon, Department of Hand Surgery, Bienville Orthopaedic Specialists, Gautier, Mississippi

NORFLEET B. THOMPSON, MD
Department of Orthopaedic Surgery and Biomedical Engineering, University of Tennessee-Campbell Clinic, Memphis, Tennessee

THOMAS (QUIN) THROCKMORTON, MD
Professor, Shoulder and Elbow Surgery, Department of Orthopaedic Surgery, University of Tennessee-Campbell Clinic, Memphis, Tennessee

JOHN C. WEINLEIN, MD
Department of Orthopaedic Surgery, University of Tennessee-Campbell Clinic, Regional One Health, Memphis, Tennessee

CONTENTS

Preface: Outpatient Surgery　　xv
Frederick M. Azar

Knee and Hip Reconstruction
Patrick C. Toy and William M. Mihalko

Outpatient Total Knee Arthroplasty: Are We There Yet? (Part 1)　　1
Andrew Krause, Zain Sayeed, Mouhanad El-Othmani, Vinay Pallekonda,
William M. Mihalko, and Khaled J. Saleh

Recent trends in total joint care have moved toward outpatient surgery. Total knee arthroplasty (TKA) remains a definitive management for end-stage osteoarthritis and has experienced increased utilization over the past several decades. The method by which surgeons conduct outpatient total knee procedures has yet to be fully elucidated, as different institutions report different experiences from their pathways. This article discusses current data and recommendations for implementing successful TKA and unicompartmental knee arthroplasty outpatient protocols. Specifically, this article provides information regarding cost reduction, patient selection criteria, and preoperative medical optimization.

Outpatient Total Knee Arthroplasty: Are We There Yet? (Part 2)　　7
Andrew Krause, Zain Sayeed, Mouhanad El-Othmani, Vinay Pallekonda,
William M. Mihalko, and Khaled J. Saleh

The method by which surgeons conduct outpatient total knee procedures has yet to be fully elucidated. Literature demonstrates different experiences from various care protocols in place across the nation. This article reviews current recommendations for implementing successful total knee arthroplasty (TKA) and unicompartmental knee arthroplasty outpatient protocols. Specifically, information regarding anesthesia and analgesia modalities, perioperative care, operative technique, and postoperative care within outpatient TKA pathways is discussed.

Total Hip Arthroplasty in the Outpatient Setting: What You Need to Know (Part 1)　　17
Zain Sayeed, Leila Abaab, Mouhanad El-Othmani, Vinay Pallekonda,
William M. Mihalko, and Khaled J. Saleh

The method by which surgeons conduct outpatient total hip arthroplasty (THA) procedures has yet to be fully standardized. Careful examination of components involved in the preoperative phase of outpatient hip arthroplasty procedures may lead to improved outcomes. This article discusses methods for implementing successful outpatient THA protocols. Specifically, it reviews information regarding patient selection criteria, preoperative education, and preoperative medical optimization.

Total Hip Arthroplasty in the Outpatient Setting: What You Need to Know (Part 2)　　27
Zain Sayeed, Leila Abaab, Mouhanad El-Othmani, Vinay Pallekonda,
William M. Mihalko, and Khaled J. Saleh

The intraoperative and postoperative phases of outpatient total hip arthroplasty (THA) vary by institution and surgeon. An understanding of an evidence-based approach to enhancing the intraoperative and postoperative phases of the care continuum is warranted to offer high-value care to outpatient candidates. This article discusses methods for implementing successful outpatient THA protocols. Specifically, it reviews information regarding anesthesia and analgesia modalities, intraoperative considerations, and postoperative rehabilitation amenable to outpatient THA.

Impact of Outpatient Total Joint Replacement on Postoperative Outcomes　　35
Danielle Lovett-Carter, Zain Sayeed, Leila Abaab, Vinay Pallekonda,
William M. Mihalko, and Khaled J. Saleh

> Total joint arthroplasty (TJA) has demonstrated tremendous benefits to patients
> with osteoarthritis. Health care reform has influenced surgeons to optimize TJA
> care pathways as well as playing a role in the formation of outpatient TJA protocols.
> Understanding the outcomes of outpatient TJA is imperative to surgical predicate
> decision making. The aim of this article was to compare outcomes of outpatient
> TJA patients to standard-stay inpatients. Postoperative outcomes assessed include
> pain, complications, readmissions, reoperation, patient satisfaction, and cost.

Trauma
John C. Weinlein and Michael J. Beebe

The Role of Implant Removal in Orthopedic Trauma　　45
Eric A. Barcak, Michael J. Beebe, and John C. Weinlein

> Although implant removal is common after orthopedic trauma, indications for
> removal remain controversial. There are few data in the literature to allow
> evidence-based decision making. The risk of complications from implant
> removal must be weighed against the possible benefits and the likelihood of
> improving the patient's symptoms.

Pediatrics
Jeffrey R. Sawyer

Outpatient Pediatric Orthopedic Surgery　　55
Daniel J. Miller, Susan E. Nelson, Apurva S. Shah, Theodore J. Ganley, and
John (Jack) M. Flynn

> Outpatient surgery refers to a surgical procedure that is performed without an
> overnight stay in a hospital. Outpatient surgery is associated with decreased
> individual and societal costs while achieving equivalent health outcomes and
> excellent patient satisfaction. Successful outpatient pediatric surgery is predi-
> cated on appropriate patient selection, adequate pain control, thorough pre-
> operative education, and close clinical follow-up. Continuous research in
> quality, value, and patient safety are needed to ensure that this practice con-
> tinues in as safe and efficient a manner as possible.

Hand and Wrist
Benjamin M. Mauck and James H. Calandruccio

Use of Wide-awake Local Anesthesia No Tourniquet in Hand and Wrist Surgery　　63
Murphy M. Steiner and James H. Calandruccio

> WALANT (wide-awake local anesthesia no tourniquet) appears to be a safe and
> effective anesthesia technique for many hand and wrist surgeries. Patient satis-
> faction is high because of the avoidance of preoperative testing and hospital
> admission. Postoperative recovery is rapid, and procedures can be done in
> outpatient settings, resulting in substantial savings in time and money.

Hand Surgery in the Ambulatory Surgery Center　　69
Norfleet B. Thompson and James H. Calandruccio

> Outpatient surgery, especially in freestanding ambulatory surgery centers (ASCs),
> provides a safe, cost-effective option for a variety of surgical procedures and has
> become the preferred choice over inpatient and hospital-based outpatient sur-
> gery for most hand and wrist procedures. Complication rates after ASC hand sur-
> gery are low (0.2%–2.5%). Patient dissatisfaction with ASC surgery is primarily
> associated with postoperative nausea and vomiting and inadequate pain control.

Shoulder and Elbow
Thomas (Quin) Throckmorton

Outpatient Shoulder Arthroplasty   73
Tyler J. Brolin and Thomas (Quin) Throckmorton

Health care policy makers have placed increased attention on the cost of health care, making outpatient joint arthroplasty an attractive alternative to routine hospital admission. Recent studies have shown outpatient shoulder arthroplasty is a safe and cost-effective alternative to inpatient shoulder arthroplasty. Proper patient selection, patient education, effective pain management strategies, and attention to intraoperative blood loss are keys in the success of outpatient shoulder arthroplasty.

Pain Management Strategies in Shoulder Arthroplasty   81
Jason L. Codding and Charles L. Getz

Pain control in total shoulder arthroplasty demands a multidisciplinary approach with collaboration among patients, surgeon, and anesthetist. A multimodal approach with preemptive medication, regional blockade, local anesthetics, and a combination of acetaminophen, nonsteroidal anti-inflammatory drugs, tramadol, and gabapentinoids postoperatively leads to pain control and patient satisfaction. Assessment of patients' expectations constitutes a vital aspect of the preoperative patient evaluation. Educating and psychologically preparing patients reduces postoperative pain. Patients with anxiety and depression, preoperative narcotic use, and medical comorbidities are at an increased risk for suboptimal pain control. Minimizing narcotic use decreases opioid-related adverse effects and facilitates productive rehabilitation efforts.

The Role of Superior Capsule Reconstruction in Rotator Cuff Tears   93
Paul Sethi and Wm. Grant Franco

Massive, irreparable rotator cuff disease is a challenging problem to treat, especially in the younger active patient. This condition allows the deltoid to generate anterosuperior translation and shoulder dysfunction. Ideally, this dysfunction may be improved with rotator cuff repair. However, in the setting of irreparable rotator cuff disease, normal function is challenging to restore. Superior capsule reconstruction theoretically improves function by recentering the humeral head and improving glenohumeral kinematics. This restoration of stability results in a stable fulcrum, and may allow the deltoid and remaining cuff to function more effectively.

Foot and Ankle
Clayton C. Bettin and Benjamin J. Grear

Outpatient Management of Ankle Fractures   103
Charles Qin, Robert G. Dekker II, Mia M. Helfrich, and Anish R. Kadakia

Interest in outpatient orthopedic surgery has been fueled by provider desire to control costs and development of rapid recovery protocols. Open reduction and internal fixation (ORIF) is a commonly elected treatment strategy for ankle fracture that may be performed in an outpatient setting. Lessons on cost-savings of the outpatient model in orthopedics can be learned in total joint replacement and spine surgery. Moreover, in properly selected patients, outpatient ORIF has been shown to be comparably safe. Reasons for admission of the surgically managed patient with ankle fractures, including concern for surgical delay and additional social factors, warrant further investigation.

Current Ultrasound Application in the Foot and Ankle   **109**
Nahum Michael Beard and Robert Patrick Gousse

This article is a comprehensive review of the current utilizations of ultrasound in the treatment of orthopedic conditions of the foot and ankle. It reviews the diagnostic and interventional applications to commonly encountered lower-extremity ailments, including plantar fasciosis, tendinosis, and peripheral nerve disorders. It also outlines minimally invasive ultrasound-guided procedures and emerging therapies as alternatives to current treatments. These emerging therapies can be used to assist surgeons and provide options for patients needing intervention. Techniques such as hydrodissection, injection, aspiration, tenotomy, and fasciotomy are discussed, giving readers insight into different treatment modalities and options to help manage their patients.

OUTPATIENT SURGERY

FORTHCOMING ISSUES

April 2018
Evidence-Based Medicine
Michael J. Beebe, Clayton C. Bettin,
James H. Calandruccio, Benjamin J. Grear,
Benjamin M. Mauck, William M. Mihalko,
Jeffrey R. Sawyer, Thomas (Quin) Throckmorton,
Patrick C. Toy, and John C. Weinlein, *Editors*

July 2018
Obesity
Michael J. Beebe, Clayton C. Bettin,
James H. Calandruccio, Benjamin J. Grear,
Benjamin M. Mauck, William M. Mihalko,
Jeffrey R. Sawyer, Thomas (Quin) Throckmorton,
Patrick C. Toy, and John C. Weinlein, *Editors*

October 2018
Quality, Value, and Patient Safety in
Orthopedic Surgery
Michael J. Beebe, Clayton C. Bettin, James H.
Calandruccio, Benjamin J. Grear, Benjamin M.
Mauck, William M. Mihalko, Jeffrey R. Sawyer,
Thomas (Quin) Throckmorton, Patrick C. Toy, and
John C. Weinlein, *Editors*

RECENT ISSUES

October 2017
Perioperative Pain Management
Clayton C. Bettin, James H. Calandruccio,
Benjamin J. Grear, Benjamin M. Mauck, Jeffrey R.
Sawyer, Patrick C. Toy, and John C. Weinlein,
Editors

July 2017
Orthobiologics
James H. Calandruccio, Benjamin J. Grear,
Benjamin M. Mauck, Jeffrey R. Sawyer,
Patrick C. Toy, and John C. Weinlein, *Editors*

April 2017
Infection
James H. Calandruccio, Benjamin J. Grear,
Benjamin M. Mauck, Jeffrey R. Sawyer,
Patrick C. Toy, and John C. Weinlein, *Editors*

ISSUE OF RELATED INTEREST

Physical Medicine and Rehabilitation Clinics of North America, August 2016 (Vol. 27, No. 3)
Outpatient Ultrasound-Guided Musculoskeletal Techniques
Evan Peck, *Editor*
Available at: http://www.pmr.theclinics.com/

PREFACE

Outpatient Surgery

Over the last several years, a number of orthopedic procedures traditionally done as inpatient procedures in a standard hospital setting have transitioned to outpatient procedures done in "one-day" surgery suites or free-standing ambulatory surgery centers (ASCs). This transition requires careful planning and consideration on multiple levels. The authors of this issue of *Orthopedic Clinics of North America* have provided valuable guidelines and recommendations for ensuring patient safety and obtaining satisfactory outcomes.

With the current emphasis on efficiency and cost-effectiveness in health care, many surgeons and patients are finding the ASC to be a viable option for total joint arthroplasty. In a two-part review, Dr Krause and colleagues present in-depth coverage of the details of outpatient total knee arthroplasty, including patient selection, medical optimization, operative technique, and postoperative care. Dr Sayeed and colleagues provide similar information for outpatient total hip arthroplasty in their reviews, and Drs Brolin and Throckmorton and Codding and Getz outline keys to success in outpatient total shoulder arthroplasty.

Although implant removal is a frequent outpatient procedure after orthopedic surgery, its indications remain controversial. Drs Barcak, Beebe, and Weinlein describe commonly cited indications for, as well as benefits and complications of, implant removal after fractures. Outpatient treatment of acute fractures of the foot and ankle is discussed by Dr Qin and colleagues, with emphasis on the few reports of outcomes, safety, and cost savings as well as the need for larger, prospective studies to clarify these issues. The use of ultrasound to identify other foot and ankle disorders that can be effectively treated with outpatient procedures such as injection, aspiration, tenotomy, and fasciotomy is thoroughly described by Drs Beard and Gousse, who also provide insight into innovative treatment options.

Many hand and wrist procedures have commonly been done on an outpatient basis, but the availability and efficiency of ASCs have made them the preferred choice over hospital-based outpatient surgery for many surgeons. Drs Thompson and Calandruccio report the safety and cost-effectiveness of outpatient hand and wrist surgery done in the ASC. In a related review, Drs Steiner and Calandruccio describe the use of WALANT (wide-awake local anesthesia no tourniquet) and discuss how its use has made outpatient hand and wrist more appealing. Another upper extremity operation that has been proven to be effective and safe in the ASC is capsular reconstruction for rotator cuff tears. Drs Sethi and Franco describe their technique and report their results.

Finally, Dr Miller and colleagues discuss the expanding role of ASCs in pediatric orthopedic surgery, with emphasis on appropriate patient selection, adequate pain control, thorough preoperative education of patients and caregivers, and patient safety.

This collection of reports from surgeons with experience and expertise in outpatient orthopedic procedures, especially those done in ASCs, provides a framework for decision making in the choice between inpatient and outpatient surgery. We hope it will be helpful in your practice to maintain high-quality patient care and safety, while achieving efficiency and cost-effectiveness.

Frederick M. Azar, MD
Campbell Clinic, Inc
University of Tennessee–Campbell Clinic
Department of Orthopaedic Surgery &
Biomedical Engineering
1211 Union Avenue, Suite 510
Memphis, TN 38104, USA

E-mail address:
fazar@campbellclinic.com

Orthop Clin N Am 49 (2018) xv
https://doi.org/10.1016/j.ocl.2017.10.001
0030-5898/18/© 2017 Published by Elsevier Inc.

Knee and Hip Reconstruction

Outpatient Total Knee Arthroplasty
Are We There Yet? (Part 1)

Andrew Krause, MD[a], Zain Sayeed, MD, MHA[a],
Mouhanad El-Othmani, MD[a], Vinay Pallekonda, MD[b],
William Mihalko, MD, PhD[c],
Khaled J. Saleh, MD, MSc, FRCS(C), MHCM, CPE[a],*

KEYWORDS

- Outpatient total joint arthroplasty • Total knee arthroplasty • Length of stay
- Unicompartmental knee arthroplasty • Early discharge

KEY POINTS

- Patients who qualify for outpatient knee arthroplasty are generally younger than 65 year old, with a range of 45 to 80 years. Patients older than 75 years have been found to have a higher risk of postoperative falls, knee stiffness, pain, and urinary retention, and an increased readmission risk within 1 year of surgery.
- A key part of improving outcomes, reducing costs, and improving patients' overall health status is correlated with the level of patient activation.
- Risk factors for infection include malnutrition, anemia, obesity, diabetes, alcohol or intravenous (IV) drug use, corticosteroid use, chronic liver disease, post-traumatic arthritis, prior surgery, and greater severity of comorbidities.

INTRODUCTION

The rapidly growing rate of total knee arthroplasty (TKA) performed each year is related to its success in improving function, correcting deformities, and relieving pain for patients with severe osteoarthritis (OA) of the knee. As the population of the United States continues to increase and life expectancy becomes longer, more patients will seek surgical treatment of their knees. Approximately 700,000 knee replacement procedures are performed annually in the United States. This number is projected to increase to 3.48 million procedures per year by 2030.[1] Performing TKA as an outpatient surgery has continued to increase in popularity over the past decade among both patients and surgeons.[2]

Previously, most providers and patients thought a multiple-day hospital stay was needed postoperatively for total joint replacements because of the pain, limited mobility, and infection risks. There has been a trend of earlier and safer patient discharges following total joint arthroplasty (TJA) over the past 20 years. The average length of stay (LOS) after a TJA has decreased from 9 to 4 days.[3,4] Several studies have shown that shorter LOS and outpatient arthroplasty do not increase the risk of adverse events (AEs) or complications.[3,5–7]

Funding Sources: No additional funding sources were used for this article.
Conflicts of Interest: No conflicts of interest are evident for authors of this article.
[a] Department of Orthopaedics, Detroit Medical Center, 4201 St Antoine Street, Detroit, MI 48201, USA; [b] Department of Anesthesiology – NorthStar Anesthesia at Detroit Medical Center, 4201 St Antoine Street, Detroit, MI 48201, USA; [c] Campbell Clinic Department of Orthopaedic Surgery & Biomedical Engineering University of Tennessee, 956 Court Avenue, Memphis, TN 32116, USA
* Corresponding author.
E-mail address: kjsaleh@gmail.com

Orthop Clin N Am 49 (2018) 1–6
http://dx.doi.org/10.1016/j.ocl.2017.08.002

Shorter LOS after TKA is a result of accelerated clinical pathways, improved pain management protocols, minimally invasive surgery, aggressive rehabilitation, and increased information available for patients and their accompaniers. The most common reasons patients report being hesitant for an early discharge are fear of pain, a slower recovery, complications, and being dependent on someone else. Once these concerns are addressed, most patients would rather recover at home instead of prolonging their stay in the hospital.[8] Patient satisfaction surveys scores have also been shown to be higher at the time of discharge with same-day discharges.[6]

This article will discuss current data and recommendations for implementing a successful TKA and unicompartmental knee arthroplasty (UKA) outpatient protocols. It will provide information regarding patient selection criteria, preoperative medical optimization, perioperative analgesia, intraoperative techniques for TKA and UKA, accelerated care pathways, rehabilitation, and discharge protocols.

COST REDUCTION IN OUTPATIENT TOTAL KNEE ARTHROPLASTY

In 2014, more than 400,000 Medicare patients received a hip or knee replacement, costing the government more than $7 billion for the hospitalizations alone. The average Medicare cost per joint for the surgery, hospitalization, and recovery is between $16,500 and $33,000.[9] Medicare pays for approximately 55% of all TKAs in the United States.[3]

These high costs have caused both surgeons and patients to look for more affordable ways to perform TJA. Outpatient arthroplasty offers a significantly reduced cost for episode of care when compared with inpatient arthroplasty.

Two of the most effective ways to reduce the cost of TKA is to shorten the LOS and to minimize complications.[3] Repicci and Eberle evaluated the reduction in cost between a 3- to 4-day hospital stay to same-day discharge and estimated a $9000 difference ($16,000 vs $7000, respectively).[10] Lovald and colleagues[3] evaluated the cost of a TKA among a sample of Medicare patients from 1997 to 2009 who were discharged within 23 hours of their surgery, discharged within 1 to 2 days, or discharged within 3 to 4 days. At a 2-year follow up, the outpatient group and 1- to 2-day stay group had costs $8527 and $1967 lower than the 3- to 4-day stay group, respectively.

During the 1990s, cost reduction programs were developed to decrease the hospital cost of TKA. Implementation of a clinical pathway and a knee-implant standardization program at the Lahey Clinic was associated with a reduction in the average LOS in the hospital from 6.79 days in 1992, to 4.16 days in 1995. The cohort of patients in 1992 and 1995 both had high patient satisfaction, low pain scores and high clinical scores at 8 and 5 years postoperatively.[11] Hospital costs were reduced 19% with the implementation of the clinical pathway and the knee-implant standardization program after adjusting for inflation.[11]

Rates of readmission for all causes within 30 days of discharge is 1 of the safety and cost-effective measures the Affordable Care Act is using to award financial incentives or penalties. A shorter length of hospital stay is considered safe and cost-effective as long as the rate of 30-day readmissions is not increased.

Balancing the cost savings of outpatient with patient outcomes is particularly relevant with the passage of the Medicare Access and Children's Health Insurance Program (CHIP) Reauthorization Act (MACRA) in 2015. This legislation shifted US health care from a volume-based to value-based payment system. Starting April 1, 2016, the Care for Joint Replacement (CJR) model started assessing the effect of bundled payments for the care of procedures such as hip or knee replacements.[12]

This is in contrast to the previous Centers for Medicare & Medicaid Services (CMS) Bundled Payment for Care Improvement (BPCI) initiative. CJR calculates each hospital's target price per 90-day episode of care by evaluating the spending data at each institution, as well as the average spending price for other hospitals in the region. Depending on their performance, participating institutions either receive bonuses from Medicare or are required to repay Medicare for a portion of the episode of spending.[12]

Currently information regarding expansion of CJR to cover outpatient TJA for Medicare patients in the future is limited. Several private insurance companies have started bundling payments to give a single payment whether a TJA is done inpatient or outpatient. Reducing the length of stay after a TKA will decrease the cost hospitals have to pay for each patient. Because shorter LOS creates a larger net gain for hospitals, it is financially advantageous for hospitals to maximize the number of patients who can be safely discharged within 23 hours of their surgery.

Under the CJR model, hospitals carry most of the risk for the value of care, as opposed to BPCI, where management firms, hospitals, and physician practices may be evaluated by CMS. By 2019, physicians can choose to be under the merit-based incentive payment systems (MIPS), where their reimbursement will be based on performance, or alternative payment models (APMs). Part of the MIPS performance measurement includes quality (30%) and clinical practice improvement (15%). The quality includes 30-day readmission rates, LOS, complications, and hospital-acquired conditions. The clinical practice improvement includes care coordination and patient safety. In order to maintain high reimbursement under the MIPS system, providers must be able to maximize the quality of care patients receive and maximize the coordination of care.[12]

PATIENT SELECTION CRITERIA

Patient selection for outpatient joint arthroplasty (OJA) is critical to minimize AEs and readmissions.[13] There is currently a lack of randomized controlled studies assessing patients' fitness for OJA. All patients should be primary arthroplasty patients without a history of knee surgery.

Outpatient arthroplasty literature has demonstrated that patients who qualify for OJA are generally younger than 65 years old, with a range of 45 to 80 years.[6] Patients older than 75 years have been found to have a higher risk of postoperative falls, knee stiffness, pain, and urinary retention, and an increased readmission risk within 1 year of surgery.[13,14]

In order to properly implement outpatient arthroplasty pathways, it is important to create inclusion and exclusion criteria. Simultaneous bilateral TKA, surgery performed for fracture, and orthopedic complexity (eg, bone loss or retained hardware) should all exclude patients from outpatient surgery.[2] Simultaneous bilateral TKA carries an increased risk of serious cardiac complications, pulmonary emboli and mortality, when compared with staged bilateral or unilateral surgery.[15] The risks of these complications are too high to perform these surgeries in outpatient surgery centers. The level of support to properly treat these complications is not comparable to inpatient hospitals.

Kort and colleagues[13] recommended that patients with uncontrolled (hemoglobin A1C >7.0%) diabetes mellitus (type I or II), a body mass index (BMI) greater than 30 kg/m^2, bleeding disorders, American Society of Anesthesiologist (ASA) scores greater than II, poorly controlled cardiac (eg, heart failure, arrhythmia) or pulmonary (eg, embolism, respiratory failure) comorbidities, chronic opioid consumptions, functional neurologic impairments, chronic or end-stage renal disease, and/or reduced preoperative cognitive capacity should be excluded from outpatient joint surgeries. Expert opinion of exclusion criteria also includes severe mobility disorders, voiding difficulties or preoperative use of urologic medications, and practical issues.

Obesity has a negative effect on outcomes after TKA. In a 2012 meta-analysis of 20 studies, patients with a BMI of at least 30 kg/m^2 demonstrated increased rates of infection (odds ratio [OR] 1.90, 95% confidence interval [CI] 1.47–2.47) and revision for any reason compared to patients with BMIs less than 30 kg/m^2.[16] This can make qualifying for outpatient surgery difficult, as approximately 50% of TKA patients are obese. Berger and colleagues[8] excluded patients who had a BMI greater than 40 kg/m^2 or with at least 3 significant medical conditions. Patients were also excluded if they were within 1 year of a myocardial infarction or pulmonary embolism, or on anticoagulation. They did not exclude patients living alone.

Uncontrolled diabetes mellitus is associated with higher rates of stroke, urinary tract infection (UTI), ileus, wound infections, postoperative hemorrhage, and death. If a surgeon determines that a diabetic patient is fit for outpatient knee arthroplasty, he or she should attempt to operate on diabetics earlier in the day in order to better control their glucose levels and minimize the risk of postoperative complications.[17]

Patients with moderate-to-severe chronic kidney disease have double the risk of mortality and a higher risk of postoperative AEs compared to patients without kidney disease.[3,13] Kolisek and colleagues[4] excluded patients if they had any history of diabetes, myocardial infarction, stroke, congestive heart failure, venous thromboembolism, cardiac arrhythmia, respiratory failure, or chronic pain requiring regular opioid medications. Chronic opioid consumption increases the difficulty in postoperative pain control.[4]

Patients with ischemic heart disease have not been shown to have higher rates of AEs following OJA.[18] However, myocardial ischemia has been shown to prolong discharge times in patients after TJA.[13,19] Cardiovascular-related major systemic AEs and deaths after TJA include 42% to 75% of the total.[17] Patients who receive bare-metal coronary stents should wait 4 to 6 weeks to have an elective total joint surgery. Moreover, patients should wait 4 weeks after balloon angioplasty and 12 months after placement of a drug-eluting stent.[17] Patients who have had a balloon angioplasty or stent should stay on aspirin during the perioperative period. Patients with a stent may also be on clopidogrel during the perioperative period, as studies have shown there is only a small increased risk of bleeding and hematoma formation. Pacemakers and defibrillators should be tested within 3 to 6 months of surgery.[17]

Acute exacerbation of chronic obstructive pulmonary disease (COPD) should delay elective TJA.[17] Patients with COPD have a 2.7 to 4.7 times increased risk of postoperative pulmonary complications after TJA.[20] Preoperative spirometry should be tested on all COPD patients, and arterial blood gas analysis should be performed for patients with moderate-to-severe COPD. If patients have a predicted postoperative (ppo) forced expiratory volume in 1 second (FEV_1) less than 40% or a carbon dioxide diffusing capacity of the lung less than 40%, aerobic capacity testing can be done to determine operative fitness. Patients who cannot climb 3 flights (54 steps) due to breathing difficulties are not recommended for surgery. Maximum oxygen consumption (Vo_{2max}) can be used for patients who cannot be tested using stairs for other reasons. Vo_{2max} less than 15 mL/kg/min or ppo Vo_{2max} <10 mL/kg/min should not be considered for surgery.[21]

PATIENT EDUCATION AND SOCIAL OPTIMIZATION

Preoperative Education Programs for Outpatient Total Knee Arthroplasty

Patients and their coach, who will support the patient after the surgery, are encouraged to attend an educational class to learn what to expect before, during, and after the surgery. They should receive clinical training from their surgeon, nurses, and physical therapists about issues and challenges they may face. A key part of improving outcomes, reducing costs, and improving patients' overall health status is correlated with the level of patient activation. Patient activation is individuals' proficiency in managing their own health care. Low levels of patient activation have been shown to have higher present-day and future health care costs. Alternatively, higher activation is correlated with increased confidence of patients to perform tasks on their own and to manage their own care at home. All members of the health care team need to work with patients to improve their confidence in managing their own care. Improving activation leads to shorter LOS, reduced costs, and improved outcomes after

surgery.[22] Patients who feel more proficient in managing their perioperative and postoperative care are more likely to qualify for outpatient surgery and have improved outcomes.

Family Anxiety

Controlling the anxiety level in the patient's family, friends, and other accompaniers has been shown to help reduce the patient's anxiety pre-, peri-, and postoperatively. Perioperative education is effective at preventing and reducing anxiety for both the patient and his or her support members. Surgical waiting rooms can provide pamphlets of procedure information, information cards, and status boards to help reduce anxiety for the patient's accompaniers. The information cards contain material regarding surgical durations, important telephone numbers, and how to obtain room assignments. Status calls regarding the patient's status, the stage of the procedure, and when the patient will be moved from recovery to his or her room have all been shown to reduce support family members' anxiety. Information delivered in person has been shown to reduce the anxiety of the patient's accompanier to a greater extent than calls if possible. Reducing the level of anxiety among accompaniers of patients minimizes the level of anxiety in the patient and has been shown to improve patient outcomes.[23]

MEDICAL OPTIMIZATION

In order to improve outcomes and minimize AEs, each patient considered for outpatient arthroplasty should be optimized regarding his or her medical conditions, nutritional status, and medications before surgery. A primary care provider should medically clear each patient before surgery. Patients undergoing total hip or knee arthroplasty with a preoperative lymphocyte count less than 1500 cells/mm have a 3 to 5 times higher frequency of a major wound complication; patients with an albumin level less than 3.5 g/dL have a 7 times greater frequency.[24,25] Transferrin levels less than 200 mg/dL and prealbumin levels less than 22.5 mg/dL are correlated with significantly higher complication rates.[17] Patients with a hemoglobin level less than 13 g/dL are 4 to 5.6 times more likely to need a blood transfusion compared with an Hb level between 13 and 15 g/dL. Because postoperative blood transfusions increase the risk of infection, it is recommended that anemic patients receive multivitamins and iron supplements to optimize their hemoglobin level before surgery.[17]

It is recommended that aspirin and nonsteroidal anti-inflammatory drugs (NSAIDs) should be stopped at least 1 week prior to surgery. Warfarin should be discontinued 3 to 5 days before surgery, and patients should have a normal prothrombin time (PT) and international normalized ratio (INR) at the time of surgery. Patients with mechanical heart valves should be bridged with low molecular weight heparin or preoperatively hospitalized to receive heparin. Heparin should be discontinued 6 hours preoperatively, and a partial thromboplastin time (PTT) should be checked. Patients should be off other antibiotics for 48 hours prior to surgery.

Oral hypoglycemic medications should be held the day of surgery. Obstructive sleep apnea is associated with higher rates of complications and longer LOS, but screening and management can reduce these rates.[17]

Risk factors for infection include malnutrition, anemia, obesity, diabetes, alcohol or intravenous (IV) drug use, corticosteroid use, chronic liver disease, post-traumatic arthritis, prior surgery, and greater severity of comorbidities. Additionally, malnutrition is associated with longer postoperative discharge times and a 5 to 7 times higher risk of developing a major wound complication after TJA.[17] Testing for zinc and vitamin D is recommended 3 weeks preoperatively, and levels should be optimized if either of these levels is not within normal ranges.

Patients with a history of alcohol abuse should abstain for at least 1 month before surgery. This significantly decreases morbidity after surgery including the risk of dislocation. Alcohol abusive patients should be screened for liver disease and malnutrition.[17] Smoking cessation for 6 to 8 weeks before surgery decreases the risk of infection, hematoma, and wound complications.[17] Abstaining for at least 4 weeks before surgery can decrease postoperative complications.[20] Patients with a history of IV drug use should be clean for at least 2 years before a TJA to decrease their risk of joint infection.

SUMMARY

This article discussed the current data and recommendations regarding implementing successful TKA outpatient protocols. Specifically, it provided information regarding cost reduction, patient selection criteria, and preoperative medical optimization. Outpatient TKA will likely be considered the gold standard in select patients within the coming years. It is imperative that the adult reconstructive community understands the benefits and pitfalls associated with implementing such procedures, and also for which patients the pathway may be amenable.

REFERENCES

1. Kurtz S, Ong K, Lau E, et al. Projections of primary and revision hip and knee arthroplasty in the United States from 2005 to 2030. J Bone Joint Surg Am 2007;89(4):780–5.
2. Meneghini RM, Ziemba-Davis M, Ishmael MK, et al. Safe selection of outpatient joint arthroplasty patients with medical risk stratification: the "outpatient arthroplasty risk assessment score". J Arthroplasty 2017;32(8):2325–31.
3. Lovald ST, Ong KL, Malkani AL, et al. Complications, mortality, and costs for outpatient and short-stay total knee arthroplasty patients in comparison to standard-stay patients. J Arthroplasty 2014;29(3):510–5.
4. Kolisek FR, McGrath MS, Jessup NM, et al. Comparison of outpatient versus inpatient total knee arthroplasty. Clin Orthop Relat Res 2009;467(6): 1438–42.
5. Teeny SM, York SC, Benson C, et al. Does shortened length of hospital stay affect total knee arthroplasty rehabilitation outcomes? J Arthroplasty 2005;20(7 Suppl 3):39–45.
6. Berger RA, Kusuma SK, Sanders SA, et al. The feasibility and perioperative complications of outpatient knee arthroplasty. Clin Orthopaedics Relat Res 2009;467(6):1443–9.
7. Isaac D, Falode T, Liu P, et al. Accelerated rehabilitation after total knee replacement. Knee 2005; 12(5):346–50.
8. Berger RA, Sanders S, Gerlinger T, et al. Outpatient total knee arthroplasty with a minimally invasive technique. J Arthroplasty 2005;20(7 Suppl 3):33–8.
9. Comprehensive care for joint replacement (CJR) model. 2015; Available at: https://www.cms.gov/Newsroom/MediaReleaseDatabase/Fact-sheets/2015-Fact-sheets-items/2015-11-16.html. Accessed April 27, 2017.
10. Repicci JA, Eberle RW. Minimally invasive surgical technique for unicondylar knee arthroplasty. J South Orthopaedic Assoc 1999;8(1):20–7 [discussion 27].
11. Healy WL, Iorio R, Ko J, et al. Impact of cost reduction programs on short-term patient outcome and hospital cost of total knee arthroplasty. J Bone Joint Surg Am 2002;84-A(3):348–53.
12. Saleh KJ, Shaffer WO. Understanding value-based reimbursement models and trends in orthopaedic health policy: an introduction to the Medicare access and chip reauthorization act (MACRA) of 2015. J Am Acad Orthop Surg 2016;24(11): e136–47.

13. Kort NP, Bemelmans YF, van der Kuy PH, et al. Patient selection criteria for outpatient joint arthroplasty. Knee Surg Sports Traumatol Arthrosc 2017; 25(9):2668–75.

14. Kort NP, Bemelmans YF, Schotanus MG. Outpatient surgery for unicompartmental knee arthroplasty is effective and safe. Knee Surg Sports Traumatol Arthrosc 2015;25(9):2659–67.

15. Restrepo C, Parvizi J, Dietrich T, et al. Safety of simultaneous bilateral total knee arthroplasty. A meta-analysis. J Bone Joint Surg Am 2007;89(6): 1220–6.

16. Kerkhoffs GM, Servien E, Dunn W, et al. The influence of obesity on the complication rate and outcome of total knee arthroplasty: a meta-analysis and systematic literature review. J Bone Joint Surg Am 2012;94(20):1839–44.

17. Ng VY, Lustenberger D, Hoang K, et al. Preoperative risk stratification and risk reduction for total joint reconstruction: AAOS exhibit selection. J Bone Joint Surg Am 2013;95(4). e191–115.

18. Lovald S, Ong K, Lau E, et al. Patient selection in outpatient and short-stay total knee arthroplasty. J Surg Orthop Adv 2014;23(1):2–8.

19. Bass AR, Rodriguez T, Hyun G, et al. Myocardial ischaemia after hip and knee arthroplasty: incidence and risk factors. Int Orthopaedics 2015; 39(10):2011–6.

20. Kakar PN, Roy PM, Pant V, et al. Anesthesia for joint replacement surgery: Issues with coexisting diseases. J Anaesthesiol Clin Pharmacol 2011;27(3): 315–22.

21. Celli BR, MacNee W. Standards for the diagnosis and treatment of patients with COPD: a summary of the ATS/ERS position paper. Eur Respir J 2004; 23(6):932–46.

22. Tzeng A, Tzeng TH, Vasdev S, et al. The role of patient activation in achieving better outcomes and cost-effectiveness in patient care. JBJS Rev 2015; 3(1).

23. Wilson CJ, Mitchelson AJ, Tzeng TH, et al. Caring for the surgically anxious patient: a review of the interventions and a guide to optimizing surgical outcomes. Am J Surg 2016;212(1):151–9.

24. Greene KA, Wilde AH, Stulberg BN. Preoperative nutritional status of total joint patients. Relationship to postoperative wound complications. J Arthroplasty 1991;6(4):321–5.

25. Marin LA, Salido JA, Lopez A, et al. Preoperative nutritional evaluation as a prognostic tool for wound healing. Acta Orthopaedica Scand 2002; 73(1):2–5.

Outpatient Total Knee Arthroplasty
Are We There Yet? (Part 2)

Andrew Krause, MD[a], Zain Sayeed, MD, MHA[a],
Mouhanad El-Othmani, MD[a], Vinay Pallekonda, MD[b],
William Mihalko, MD, PhD[c],
Khaled J. Saleh, MD, MSc, FRCS(C), MHCM, CPE[a],*

KEYWORDS

- Outpatient total joint arthroplasty • Total knee arthroplasty • Length of stay
- Unicompartmental knee arthroplasty • Early discharge

KEY POINTS

- Regional anesthesia with various combinations of pain control medication has proved successful, with a combination of oxycodone hydrochloride, ketorolac, hydrocodone, and acetaminophen.
- With regard to perioperative care, it is recommended to avoid use of Foley catheterization, screen and decolonize for methicillin-resistant *Staphylococcus aureus*, and provide appropriate antibiotic dosing in a timely fashion and appropriate DVT prophylaxis with aspirin in select patients.
- Various accelerated clinical care pathways have been implemented and proved successful in enhancing postoperative outcomes. These are generally optimized when coupled with best evidence-based medical interventions, such as enhanced recovery pathways.

INTRODUCTION

Total knee arthroplasty (TKA) is considered among the most effective and successful procedures in medicine because it regains functionality and quality of life to patients. As such, the rate of performance of the procedure is expected to continue its ongoing rise to reach up to 3.48 million procedures per year by 2030, from the current rate of approximately 700,000 annual procedures.[1,2] With the recent drive toward decreasing cost of care, while simultaneously elevating quality, TKA in the outpatient setting gained popularity as a cost-efficient option in specific patient populations.[3]

As value became a topic of heightened focus in care delivery, serious efforts have been undertaken to minimize wastes and resource consumption, tackling variables that might have an impact on care-related outcomes and quality. With hospital length of stay (LOS) now considered a source of added unnecessary cost with minimal benefit, and even added risk for postoperative complications, the drive toward outpatient TKA has been reinforced and accelerated.[4,5]

The role of patient selection and global optimization in the success of performing outpatient TKA is discussed (See Khaled J. Saleh's article, "Outpatient Total Knee Arthroplasty: Are We There Yet? (Part 1)," in this issue for further details). This article focuses on perioperative care

---

Funding Sources: No additional funding sources were used for this article.
Conflicts of Interest: No conflicts of interest are evident for authors of this article.
[a] Department of Orthopaedics, Detroit Medical Center, 4201 St Antoine Street, Detroit, MI 48201, USA;
[b] Department of Anesthesiology – NorthStar Anesthesia at Detroit Medical Center, Detroit Medical Center, 4201 St Antoine Street, Detroit, MI 48201, USA; [c] Campbell Clinic Department of Orthopaedic Surgery & Biomedical Engineering University of Tennessee, 956 Court Avenue, Memphis, TN 32116, USA
* Corresponding author.
E-mail address: kjsaleh@gmail.com

requirements, pain management protocols, surgical techniques, accelerated care pathways, rehabilitation, and discharge protocols.

ANESTHESIA AND ANALGESIA MODALITIES

Preoperative and Postoperative Pain Control

Patients are typically instructed to take 10 mg of controlled-release oxycodone hydrochloride prior to coming into the hospital on the morning of their surgery. Immediately after surgery, patients often receive intramuscular ketorolac (10–15 mg) and/or oral hydrocodone (5 or 7.5 mg) plus 325 mg of acetaminophen (350 mg).[5] Preemptive management with acetaminophen or cyclooxygenase-2 selective nonsteroidal anti-inflammatory drugs (NSAIDs) is often used.

Regional Anesthesia

Regional anesthesia allows for less narcotic use, which decreases postoperative nausea and hypotension and allows for faster time to ambulation. Adductor canal and infiltration between the popliteal artery and capsule of knee blocks are becoming increasingly popular. They provide appropriate analgesia, while having muscle weakness-sparing characteristics.[6]

Memtsoudis and colleagues[7] looked at the records of 191,570 elective TKA and compared the rates of inpatient falls after surgery. The study found that 10.9% of the patients had received neuraxial anesthesia, 12.9% combined neuraxial/general anesthesia, and 76.2% had general anesthesia.

Kerr and Kohan[8] developed an intraoperative anesthetic protocol for total hip and knee arthroplasty. They used a combination of ropivacaine Hydrochloride (HCL), 2.0 mg/mL, mixed with 30-mg ketorolac tromethamine and 10 µg/mL of adrenaline (ropivicanine, ketorlac, and adrenaline [RKA] mixture). The mixture was injected into the tissues around the surgical field for pain control. This local infiltration analgesia technique allows earlier postoperative mobilization and an earlier discharge. Almost all TKAs were performed with combined spinal (3.0 mL bupivacaine 0.25%) and light general anesthesia (propofol infusion or O$_2$/N$_2$O/sevoflurane). Postoperative pain was kept at less than or equal to 3 using the numeric rating scale. Only one-third of patients required morphine for postoperative pain control. Reinjection of the same anesthetic mixture was given using a catheter that was placed just anterior to the posterior capsule on the medial side approximately 20 hours after surgery in the TKA patients; 71% of the patients were discharged home after 1 night in the hospital. Unless contraindicated, ibuprofen, 400 mg was given every 4 hours for 24 hours postoperatively.[8]

Previous studies have shown that periarticular injection (PAI) of liposomal bupivacaine provides decreased use of narcotics and shorter LOS after TKA.[9] Recent studies have shown, however, that liposomal bupivacaine may not be superior to ropivacaine PAI or femoral catheter plus sciatic nerve blocks for TKA.[10–12]

Liposomal bupivacaine has also not been shown superior to standard bupivacaine after TKA. Schroer and colleagues[13] compared pain management after TKA for patients who received 266 mg (20 mL) liposomal bupivacaine combined with 75 mg (30 mL) 0.25% bupivacaine to a control group who received 150 mg (60 mL) 0.25% bupivacaine; 58 patients received the liposomal bupivacaine and 53 patients were in the control group. Although pain score and narcotic use were similar during hospitalization for the 2 groups, the cost was significantly higher for the liposomal bupivacaine ($285 vs $2.80 for the control group).

Kuang and colleagues[11] did not recommend using liposomal bupivacaine PAI for TKA over traditional PAI methods. This study found that liposomal bupivacaine had comparable pain control and functional recovery compared with conventional PAI methods (usually 2 or more agents, such as opioids, NSAIDs, steroid hormones [eg, dexamethasone or betamethasone], and local anesthetics of amide derivatives [eg, bupivacaine or ropivacaine]), but the cost for this medication did not justify a recommendation as a long-acting analgesic for TKA. A review of recent literature references comparing liposomal bupivacaine to other analgesics is listed in Table 1.[10,12]

Both adductor canal blocks (ACBs) and femoral nerve blocks (FNBs) have been shown efficacious in reducing postoperative pain after TKA. Elkassabany and colleagues[14] showed that ACB resulted in a superior preservation of quadriceps muscle strength postoperatively from TKA compared with an FNB. ACB should facilitate earlier ambulation by avoiding quadriceps weakness. The study, however, showed no significant difference in fall risk comparing ACB and FNB on postoperative day (POD) 1 or POD 2, but it may be present in a larger study cohort. Indwelling FNB catheters prolong quadriceps dysfunction and have been associated with an increased risk of falls and adverse postoperative events.[15,16]

Local periarticular and intra-articular injection using ropivacaine, ketorolac, and epinephrine has been shown to be preferred over FNB because average postoperative pain at rest

Table 1
Executive summary of higher-level evidence comparing liposomal bupivacaine to other analgesia modalities

Authors	Objective	Level of Evidence and Study Design	Type	Findings
Kuang et al,[11] 2017	Review comparative studies regarding effectiveness of liposomal bupivacaine	Level 1 evidence – meta analysis	TKA	PAI of liposomal bupivacaine was comparable to conventional PAI methods[a] in regard to length of hospital stay ($P = .53$), ROM ($P = .28$), total opioid consumption ($P = .25$), postoperative nausea ($P = .34$), ambulation distance ($P = .07$), and visual analog scale score at 24 h ($P = .46$), 48 h ($P = .43$), and 72 h ($P = .21$). Based on the increased cost for adequate pain control, the investigators did not recommend using liposomal bupivacaine as an alternative long-acting PAI agent.
DeClaire et al,[12] 2017	Compared effectiveness of liposomal bupivacaine to ropivacaine as part of multimodal pain management in TKA	Level 1 evidence – prospective, randomized, double-blind controlled study	TKA	No significant difference between ropivacaine and liposomal bupivacaine cohorts with regard to postoperative narcotic use per hour, total narcotic use during hospital stay, time to ambulation, length of stay, or VAS scores for pain. There is no benefit in use of liposomal bupivacaine compared with ropivacaine.
Amundson et al,[10] 2017	This 3-arm, nonblinded trial randomized of 165 adults undergoing unilateral primary TKA to receive (1) femoral catheter plus sciatic nerve blocks, (2) ropivacaine-based PAI, or (3) liposomal bupivacaine-based PAI	Level 2 – nonrandomized prospective cohort study	TKA	Median maximal pain scores for patients receiving femoral catheter plus sciatic nerve blocks, ropivacaine-based PAI, or liposomal bupivacaine-based PAI on POD 0 were 0.6, 1.7, and 2.4, respectively, and on POD 1 were 2.5, 3.5, and 3.7, respectively. POD 0 median maximal and average pain scores were significantly lower for peripheral nerve block compared with both PAIs (ropivacaine: maximal −2 [−3 to −1]; average −0.8 [−1.3 to −0.2]; $P < .001$; and liposomal bupivacaine: maximal −3 [−4 to −2]; average −1.4 [−2.0 to −0.8]; $P<.001$). POD 1 median maximal pain scores were significantly lower for peripheral nerve blockade compared to liposomal bupivacaine-based PAI ($P = .016$). Liposomal bupivacaine was not found superior to ropivacaine in PAI for TKA.

[a] The conventional PAI method usually contains 2 or more antalgic agents, such as opioids (eg, morphine, fentanyl, and codeine), NSAIDs (eg, diclofenac sodium, ibuprofen, and meloxicam), steroid hormones (eg, dexamethasone and betamethasone), and local anesthetics of amide derivatives (eg, bupivacaine and ropivacaine).

was marginally better and local injection is cheaper and easier to perform. Both methods reduce the amount of postoperative opioids used.[17]

PERIOPERATIVE CARE
General Surgical Care
The use of indwelling urinary catheters or intermittent urinary catheterization as needed for TKA is controversial. A meta-analysis by Zhang and colleagues[18] compared the rates of urinary tract infections and postoperative urinary retention in patients receiving a TKA. The analysis included 9 randomized controlled trials, including 1771 patients. They found that indwelling catheters that were removed within 24 hours to 48 hours had lower rates of postoperative urinary retention and no increased risk of urinary tract infections compared with intermittent catheterization. Kerr and Kohan,[8] however, did not use a urinary catheter for any of their patients that received a primary TKA.

All patients should be screened for methicillin-resistant *Staphylococcus aureus* using a nasal swab, with preoperative decolonization treatment as needed. Cefazolin intravenous (IV) antibiotics are given within 60 minutes of the start of the surgery. Two grams are given for patients weighing less than 120 kg, and 3g are given to patients weighing greater than or equal to 120 kg. A second dose is given 4 hours after the first dose. Vancomycin, 15 mg/kg IV (maximum 2 g), or clindamycin, 900 mg IV, with a second dose 6 hours later are acceptable alternative antimicrobial agents to use alone in patients with true β-lactam allergies. If there is concern for gram-negative organisms, clindamycin or vancomycin can be added to the cefazolin if the patient is not allergic to β-lactam antibiotics. Aztreonam, gentamicin, or a single-dose of a fluoroquinolone can be added to the vancomycin or clindamycin dose if the patient is β-lactam allergic and there is a risk of gram-negative infection.[19,20]

Several studies have shown that tranexamic acid (TXA) decreases postoperative blood loss and the number of blood transfusions after TKA. The American Academy of Orthopaedic Surgeons (AAOS) recommends the use of TXA for all patients receiving TKA if there are no known contraindications.[21,22] Contraindications for injectable TXA include active intravascular clotting (including clotting in the central retinal artery/vein), subarachnoid hemorrhage, acquired defective color vision, or hypersensitivity to TXA or any components. Additionally, contraindications to oral TXA includes a history of clotting, intrinsic risk of thrombosis or

thromboembolism, or concurrent hormonal contraception therapy.[23,24]

Kerr and Kohan[8] looked at 325 patients who received either an elective hip resurfacing, primary total hip arthroplasty or primary TKA between 2005 and 2006 by a single surgeon. A tourniquet was used in 98.8% of the patients in this study. Contraindication for a tourniquet included for patients who had significant peripheral vascular disease and previous vascular surgery. The tourniquet was inflated to 300 mm Hg. It was released after implantation of the femoral and tibial components and before working on the patella to minimize ischemia time and muscle pain.[8] A thigh tourniquet should be inflated for a maximum of 120 minutes. Use of a tourniquet allows for less blood loss, better visualization, and easier implantation of cement. Zhang and colleagues[25] conducted a meta-analysis involving 16 trials and 1010 patients to determine the difference between releasing the tourniquet before or after wound closure. The review found that releasing the tourniquet before wound closure had a larger blood loss and longer operative time. The study also found releasing the tourniquet before wound closure may reduce minor complications (deep vein thrombosis [DVT]), leg swelling, wound oozing, minor wound dehiscence, superficial infection, and marginal necrosis). Therefore, the investigators recommended that the tourniquet be released prior to wound closure unless the patients had severe anemia. Olivecrona and colleagues[26] also found that the rate of complications increased if the tourniquet was inflated greater than 293 mm Hg. They also found there was a lower rate of wound complications no difference in postoperative infections and with a pressure less than or equal to 225 mm Hg compared with a cuff inflated above this pressure.

Deep Vein Thrombosis Prophylaxis
Intermittent pneumatic compression can be used for patients with a high bleeding risk or can be used in combination with other anticoagulation options. Several studies used a full-strength aspirin (325 mg) daily for 6 weeks to achieve DVT prophylaxis.[8,15] Kerr and Kohan[8] used enoxaparin initially followed by warfarin for patients with a predisposition to thrombosis or previous history of thrombosis or who would not comply with the aggressive mobilization protocol. The peak incidence of venous thromboembolic events has been found to be 16 days after a TKA.[27] The compliance with DVT prophylactic medication is close to 100% in the hospital,

whereas the compliance of thromboprophylaxis after discharge from orthopedic-related procedures drops to only approximately 20%. This large drop in compliance rates is due to a combination of arranging home care, patients' hesitancy to self-inject medications, and the cost of outpatient medications.[27] Performing the surgery inpatient ensures a longer compliance with anticoagulation medication and more aggressive mobilization as well as a closer observation by medically trained professionals for the development of thromboembolic events. Based on the authors' review of the literature, excluding patients with higher tendencies of developing DVTs or a history of thromboembolic events from having the procedures done outpatient is recommended.

TECHNIQUE AND APPROACH
Medial Parapatellar
Several approaches are used successfully for outpatient TKA. The medial parapatellar (PP) approach is the most common technique used in TKA today. The patient is placed supine with a bump under the ipsilateral hip to internally rotate the leg. This approach starts by making a midline longitudinal incision 2 cm to 5 cm above the superior pole of the patella, extending to the tibial tubercle. The medial patellar retinaculum is incised between the vastus medialis and quadriceps tendon to open the joint capsule. The infrapatellar fat pad is excised or retracted, followed by dislocating the patella and flipping it laterally. Care needs to be taken to avoid avulsing the patellar ligament off of the tibial tubercle. The knee is then flexed to 90° to gain exposure to the knee.[28]

This approaches allows an ideal exposure but also destabilizes the patella by disrupting extension of the leg at the junction of the vastus medialis and quadriceps tendon. The superior geniculate artery and infrapatellar branch of the saphenous nerve are also at risk of injury during this approach.[28]

Subvastus and Modified Subvastus
The standard subvastus (SV) approach, also called the southern approach, maintains the quadriceps tendon and blood supply to the patella. This decreases blood loss compared with a medial PP. The SV is a more demanding compared with the medial PP and can increase operative time.[29,30] In contrast to the medial PP approach, a transverse incision is made in the medial capsule at the level of the upper patella and extended down the medial side of the patellar tendon. This facilitates eversion of the patella.[30] Weinhardt and colleagues[29] compared the SV and PP approach by randomly assigning 26 patients to each group and performing a primary TKA. They found that the SV group was able to flex to 90° 4 days sooner than the PP group (mean, 7.0 vs 11.0 days). The SV group could also passively extend on day 2.2 compared with day 7.7 in the PP group. The earlier recovery of quadriceps strength and less postoperative pain could help shorter discharge times for outpatient TKA.

Jung and colleagues[30] compared a modified SV to a standard medial PP. This study involved 26 patients (bilateral TKA 28 cases and unilateral TKA 12 cases). In the bilateral TKA patients, a modified SV was used on 1 knee and a medial PP on the other. A total of 19 cases were in the PP group and 21 cases in the modified SV group.

In addition to the standard SV technique, a transverse incision was made 1 cm to 2 cm from the insertion of the vastus medialis. This modification was used because patellar eversion is more difficult in muscular and obese patients and this small incision makes eversion of the patella significantly easier. This technique allows for a smaller skin incision compared with a standard SV approach. The investigators recommend avoiding this technique in obese patients with substantial patella baja.[30]

Patients who underwent the modified SV approach were able to straight leg raise an average of 1.7 days sooner than patients who underwent the medial PP approach (0.5 days vs 2.2 days). Knee flexion and range of motion (ROM) were also better up to POD 10 with the modified SV. In a subjective postoperative evaluation 3 years after surgery, 11 of 14 patients preferred the knee treated by the modified SV due to less pain and better functional activity. Vastus medialis muscle strength was not quantified during follow-up in this study.[30]

Minimally Invasive Total Knee Arthroplasty
Minimally invasive surgeries are proposed to minimize complications, improve timing of muscle strength return, and minimize pain and have been proposed to allow for earlier discharges after TKA. Berger and colleagues[31] used a minimally invasive incision in the capsule from the joint line to the superior pole of the patella without violating the quadriceps muscle or tendon. The mean incision was 9.1 cm long; 48 patients (96%) were discharged the same day. One patient was discharged the next morning and 1 patient had to stay 2 nights due to nausea. One patient had a subcutaneous infection that

did not involve the joint and resolved after irrigation and débridement at 21 days after surgery. Another patient, with a history of a bleeding gastric ulcer, had a small bleeding ulcer on POD 8. Aspirin was discontinued; the patient was managed medically and discharged without further complications. There were no other readmissions, emergency department visits, or reoperations.

At a mean follow-up of 24 months, the clinical and satisfaction scores as well as the radiographic outcomes of the patients were excellent and comparable to a matched cohort of patients who followed an inpatient protocol.[31]

Unicompartmental Knee Arthroplasty

During unicompartmental knee arthroplasty (UKA), only 1 compartment (medial, lateral or patellofemoral) of the knee is resurfaced. The preoperative protocol is the same for UKA, as described previously for TKA. The incision and operative time are both shorter during a UKA compared with a TKA. Despite having a more rapid recovery and less pain after surgery when compared with TKA, UKA is still considered by most to be an inpatient operation. Cross and Berger[32] studied 105 patients who underwent UKA as part of a rapid recovery protocol; 100% of the patients were able to be discharged home on the same day of surgery. All patients had an epidural anesthesia, and no patient required general anesthesia. No patients required readmission within the first week postoperatively.[32]

Gondusky and colleagues[15] used an effective perioperative pathway for outpatient UKA on 160 consecutive patients. Ranitidine, 150 mg orally, and midazolam, 2 mg IV, were given preoperatively. Scopolamine patches were prescribed to patients with a significant history of postoperative nausea to be applied preoperatively on the morning of surgery. Two patients received a spinal anesthetic and the rest received general anesthesia. All patients also received an ultrasound guided FNB using ropivacaine 0.5% (20 mL) and marcaine 0.5% with epinephrine (1:200,000) (10 mL) in the operating room. Intraoperative medications to control pain included IV narcotics as needed (morphine sulfate 10 mg, fentanyl 100 µg–200 µg, or meperidine 25 mg–50 mg). Standard preoperative antibiotics, usually a first-generation cephalosporin, were given before the tourniquet was inflated. A tourniquet was used for all cases. Patients received an intraoperative injection of periarticular tissues using 20 mL to 40 mL of 0.2% ropivacaine. A minimally invasive incision

was used without patellar eversion for all medial and lateral UKAs. All implants were cemented. A single drain was placed, which was removed before discharge. A knee immobilizer was applied to each patient at the end of surgery. Most patients used cold therapy, such as ice. Postoperative pain was treated with oral hydrocodone/acetaminophen and IV fentanyl (25 µg –50 µg) for breakthrough pain.

Discharge criteria required an awake, alert patient with adequate pain control, stable vital signs, and clearance by an anesthesiologist. Full weight-bearing status was allowed with PT supervision. Patients were recommended to wear their knee immobilizer for all weight-bearing activities until they were able to perform 5 straight leg raises.[15]

Preoperative PT was not routinely prescribed. Home PT began on POD 1 and was continued 3 times a week for 1 hour for 2 weeks to 3 weeks. Most patients continued outpatient PT for up to 3 months as needed based on progress. All 160 patients who were planned to be discharged on the day of surgery were able to meet discharge criteria and return home the same day as their surgery.[15]

Reilly and colleagues[33] compared an accelerated recovery protocol for UKA to a traditional protocol. The study included 41 patients, 21 randomly selected for the accelerated protocol and 20 for the standard protocol. This study found that patients in the accelerated pathway average stay was 1.5 days, whereas the standard group average was 4.3 days. There were no significant differences in outcomes between the 2 groups. The accelerated protocol cost an average of 27% less. Patient satisfaction scores were also higher at discharge compared with the routine discharge.

USE OF TECHNOLOGY (ROBOTIC VS COMPUTER-ASSISTED VS TRADITIONAL TOTAL KNEE ARTHROPLASTY)

Although the use of both robotic and computer-assisted methods for TKA has continued to increase, information regarding their utility in outpatient TKA is limited. The use of custom cutting guides for TKA has increased from 1.3% in 2009 to 6% in 2012.[34,35]

No significant difference has been found between LOS, perioperative complications, patient outcome, and satisfaction scores when comparing traditional and computer-assisted TKA (CATKA). Additionally, pain and quality-of-life outcomes have not been shown significantly different between the 2 groups.[35,36] Although computer-assisted surgery for TKA has been shown to have greater accuracy in regard to implant alignment compared with the traditional manual approach, there is a lack of evidence that this leads to better-long term results after TKA.[37] The 2016 AAOS guideline on Surgical Management of Osteoarthritis of the Knee has recommended against the use of navigation. The AAOS recommendation was based on multiple studies that found there were no significant differences in outcomes or complications.[35,36] Future practice guidelines may amend the current policy and further investigation is warranted.

Minimally invasive CATKA has been shown superior to the traditional computer-assisted approach. Khakha and colleagues[38] showed that using an incision less than 12 cm with a mini-midvastus approach CATKA had a shorter LOS (mean, 3.25 days vs 6 days) and higher Knee Society scores at up to a 2-year follow-up compared with the traditional CATKA; 40 patients were in both the minimally invasive and traditional cohorts in this study. By day 1, 93% of the minimally invasive group was able to straight leg raise compared with 30% of the traditional CATKA patients. There was no significant difference in Knee Society scores at 5 years between the 2 groups.

CARE PATHWAYS
Accelerated Clinical Pathway
Accelerated clinical pathways, also known as fast-track or rapid recovery protocols, are multimodal protocols used to expedite discharges for patients undergoing different procedures. In addition to shortening LOS, they also attempt to reduce perioperative morbidity by improving pain management and rehabilitation. These pathways require effective coordination between the multidisciplinary team, including the patient, surgeon, anesthesiologist, surgical nurse, and physiotherapist.[39] For this program to be successful in TKA, the surgical team must optimize control of postoperative nausea, pain control, prolonged urinary retention, hypotension, and patient anxiety and have a motived team of physical therapists (PTs), clinical nurses, and discharge planners.[32] Discharge planners call patients the day before surgery to make sure someone is available to take the patient home at discharge and someone to help once the patient gets home.

Kolisek and colleagues[5] compared an accelerated pathway where patients were discharged within 23 hours to a standard inpatient cohort. There were 64 patients in each cohort and the 2 groups were matched for age, gender, body mass index, and length of follow-up. At 24 months' follow-up, no one in the accelerated group had been readmitted to the hospital for complications related to the TKA.

The study compared perioperative (within 90 days of the surgery) complications, Knee Society knee and functional scores, ranges of motion, satisfaction scores, and radiographic outcomes for patients in both cohorts. Mean operative time for both inpatient and outpatient was 45 minutes. Patients discharged within 23 hours as well as the inpatients that stayed for 2 days to 3 days had similar short-term outcomes and no perioperative complications. Knee Society function scores at 24 months were an average of 86 points for both groups. The mean Knee Society knee scores were 94 for outpatient and 93 for inpatient. Mean ROM was slightly better in the outpatient group, 123° versus 121° for inpatients.[5]

Patients who were in the accelerated cohort were discharged after they demonstrated that they could eat food and drink liquid without difficulty, could ambulate with a walker, and could perform the slide and flex, tighten, extend (SAFTE) exercises and that their pain was well managed with oral medications. A home health nurse then saw these patients on the second POD and they visited a PT on POSDs 2 to 5. Patients returned for follow-up evaluations at 6 weeks, 6 months, 1 year, and then annually.[5]

The most common reasons for delayed discharges for patients in enhanced recovery pathways are pain and postoperative nausea and vomiting.[40,41] Preemptive antiemetic medications decrease postoperative nausea in the recovery phase.

Nausea prophylaxis is typically achieved with ondansetron hydrochloride, 4 mg IV, every 4 to 8 hours as needed,[5] and/or metoclopramide, 10 mg, given IV during surgery.

All these reduced pathways must ensure that there are no adverse effects on patient outcomes.

Berger and colleagues[40] found that 104 (94%) of the 111 patients who underwent a primary UKA or TKA completed by noon were discharged directly home the day of surgery. Four patients (3.6%) were readmitted and 1 patient had an emergency room visit without readmission within the first week postoperatively. Readmission rates may be slightly higher in patients discharged the same day as their surgery compared with patients that stayed in the hospital for at least day after their surgery. Patients who qualify preoperatively for outpatient total joint arthroplasty, however, have great success at being discharged within 23 hours of their surgery.

Lovald and colleagues[4] found that the rate of readmission within 90 days postoperatively for patients who had their surgery outpatient, discharged within 1 day to 2 days, within 3 to 4 days, or greater than or equal to 5 days after their surgery were 0.9%, 0.6%, 0.5%, and 0.8%, respectively. The slight increase in the readmission rates for patients discharged in less than or equal to 2 days compared with the 3-day to 4-day LOS patients highlights the risk of discharging patients earlier.

Enhanced Recovery Pathways

Enhanced recovery pathways change the previous thought of overnight fasting, to encouraging patients to drink carbohydrates up until 2 hours preoperative as well as serving food the same day as the surgery. This protocol also recommends balancing fluids during surgery rather than giving large volumes of IV fluids. These protocols have reduced hospital stays by 30% to 50%, while also reducing readmissions, complications, and costs.[42] Kerr and Kohan[8] used 2 L of Hartmann solution and 500 mL of 4% albumin intraoperatively plus an additional 2 L of Hartmann solution and 0.5 L of 4% albumin over the next 24 hours. Enhanced recovery pathways are becoming the standard of care in surgery and for total joint arthroplasty.

POSTOPERATIVE CONSIDERATIONS
Physical Therapy

Perioperative therapy is critical to proper healing after any arthroplasty; however, information regarding the timing and duration of therapy is still unclear. Improved rehabilitation after outpatient TKA has been proposed as a major contributing factor to shorter LOS and earlier ambulation.[4]

A meta-analysis by Minns Lowe and colleagues[43] showed that PT supervised functional exercise programs improve knee function and ROM in the first 3 months to 4 months postoperative compared with routine care, but no difference was found between the 1 groups at 1 year.

Patients are encouraged to start moving their feet and ankles immediately after surgery. Some surgeons use a continuous passive motion device while a patient is still in bed. Continuous passive motion devices have not been shown to be clinically advantageous to improve ROM, pain, prevention of DVTs, function, or quality of life compared with standard therapy[44]

Patients are usually able to resume normal activities within 3 weeks to 6 weeks after surgery. Isaac and colleagues[45] looked at accelerated rehabilitation protocols after TKA. Under PT supervision, patients were ambulatory within 4 hours postoperatively with the assistance of a walker. The operative leg was rested in full extension using a pillow under the heel to maintain extension and avoid flexion contractures. Physical therapy encouraged straight leg exercises. Due to institution policies, patients were only discharged once they could safely walk with crutches and climb stairs independently.

Kerr and Kohan's[8] postoperative protocol tried to mobilize all patients within 3 hours to 4 hours after surgery, followed by every 2 hours to 3 hours. A 200-mL to 300-mL fluid bolus was given before having the patient stand for the first time. Patients were encouraged to walk at least 30 meters. Patients were encouraged to walk independently with crutches, followed by self-mobilization without the crutches.[8]

Evidence regarding the utility of supervised preoperative PT is limited. Berger and colleagues[31] had patients attend a single PT session to learn gait training with crutches and a cane. Postoperatively, patients were required to independently transfer from the bed to standing and standing to the bed, stand from a chair and sit from standing, ascend and descend 1 flight of stairs, and ambulate 100 feet to be discharged.

Jones and colleagues[46] found that patients may be encouraged to engage in low to moderate intensity activities long term after a TKA because it was not shown to increase the risk of a revision arthroplasty. PT can be continued at home for 1 week to 2 weeks, at a PT office or using an exercise bike on their own.

Ko and colleagues[47] compared 1-to-1 therapy with group and home-based therapy after primary TKA. Patients were randomly assigned to complete either 12 1-to-1 therapy sessions, 12 group-based therapy sessions, or a monitored home-based program. The study involved 85 patients in the 1-to-1 sessions, 84 in the group-based sessions, and 80 patients in the home program, with patient characteristics similar across all 3 groups. The group therapy involved a 53-minute circuit with different stations that was conducted by a PT. Patients in the home monitored program attended 2 individual PT sessions, 1 at the beginning and the second 2 weeks later. At the first session, participants received an instructional DVD and booklet to keep track of their progression. Oxford Knee Scores at week 10 were 32 points, 36 points, and 34 points for the 1-to-1, group, and home-based program, respectively (best score possible of 48 points). The study also found that the 1-to-1 group was not superior to the other 2 cohorts regarding secondary outcomes (pain subscale and 6-minute walk distance) during the first year after surgery.

SUMMARY

Our article highlights the evidence-based approaches that allow the establishment and delivery of a successful outpatient TKA program. Patient-specific variables and various components of the continuum of care remain critical to elevating the value of the procedure, in terms of minimizing waste and improving postoperative outcomes. As highlighted in the second part of this article, there is no single approach that has been proved the gold standard. The general concept remains on optimizing all the different components of the continuum, starting at the surgeon's clinic until as long as needed after discharge.

REFERENCES

1. Schwarzkopf R, Brodsky M, Garcia GA, et al. Surgical and functional outcomes in patients undergoing total knee replacement with patient-specific implants compared with "off-the-shelf" implants. Orthop J Sports Med 2015;3(7). 2325967115590379.
2. Kurtz S, Ong K, Lau E, et al. Projections of primary and revision hip and knee arthroplasty in the United States from 2005 to 2030. J Bone Joint Surg Am 2007;89(4):780–5.
3. Meneghini RM, Ziemba-Davis M, Ishmael MK, et al. Safe selection of outpatient joint arthroplasty patients with medical risk stratification: the "outpatient arthroplasty risk assessment score". J Arthroplasty 2017;32(8):2325–31.
4. Lovald ST, Ong KL, Malkani AL, et al. Complications, mortality, and costs for outpatient and short-stay total knee arthroplasty patients in comparison to standard-stay patients. J Arthroplasty 2014;29(3):510–5.
5. Kolisek FR, McGrath MS, Jessup NM, et al. Comparison of outpatient versus inpatient total knee arthroplasty. Clin Orthop Relat Res 2009;467(6):1438–42.
6. Cullom C, Weed JT. Anesthetic and analgesic management for outpatient knee arthroplasty. Curr Pain Headache Rep 2017;21(5):23.
7. Memtsoudis SG, Danninger T, Rasul R, et al. Inpatient falls after total knee arthroplasty: the role of anesthesia type and peripheral nerve blocks. Anesthesiology 2014;120(3):551–63.
8. Kerr DR, Kohan L. Local infiltration analgesia: a technique for the control of acute postoperative pain following knee and hip surgery: a case study of 325 patients. Acta Orthop 2008;79(2):174–83.
9. Webb BT, Spears JR, Smith LS, et al. Periarticular injection of liposomal bupivacaine in total knee arthroplasty. Arthroplasty Today 2015;1(4):117–20.
10. Amundson AW, Johnson RL, Abdel MP, et al. A three-arm randomized clinical trial comparing continuous femoral plus single-injection sciatic peripheral nerve blocks versus periarticular injection with ropivacaine or liposomal bupivacaine for patients undergoing total knee arthroplasty. Anesthesiology 2017;126(6):1139–50.
11. Kuang MJ, Du Y, Ma JX, et al. The efficacy of liposomal bupivacaine using periarticular injection in total knee arthroplasty: a systematic review and meta-analysis. J Arthroplasty 2017;32(4):1395–402.
12. DeClaire JH, Aiello PM, Warritay OK, et al. Effectiveness of bupivacaine liposome injectable suspension for postoperative pain control in total knee arthroplasty: a prospective, randomized, double blind, controlled study. J Arthroplasty 2017;32(9S):S268–71.
13. Schroer WC, Diesfeld PG, LeMarr AR, et al. Does extended-release liposomal bupivacaine better control pain than bupivacaine after total knee arthroplasty (TKA)? a prospective, randomized clinical trial. J Arthroplasty 2015;30(9 Suppl):64–7.
14. Elkassabany NM, Antosh S, Ahmed M, et al. The risk of falls after total knee arthroplasty with the use of a femoral nerve block versus an adductor canal block: a double-blinded randomized controlled study. Anesth Analgesia 2016;122(5):1696–703.
15. Gondusky JS, Choi L, Khalaf N, et al. Day of surgery discharge after unicompartmental knee arthroplasty: an effective perioperative pathway. J Arthroplasty 2014;29(3):516–9.
16. Feibel RJ, Dervin GF, Kim PR, et al. Major complications associated with femoral nerve catheters for knee arthroplasty: a word of caution. J Arthroplasty 2009;24(6 Suppl):132–7.
17. Affas F, Nygards EB, Stiller CO, et al. Pain control after total knee arthroplasty: a randomized trial comparing local infiltration anesthesia and continuous femoral block. Acta Orthop 2011;82(4):441–7.
18. Zhang W, Liu A, Hu D, et al. Indwelling versus intermittent urinary catheterization following total joint arthroplasty: a systematic review and meta-analysis. PLoS One 2015;10(7):e0130636.
19. AlBuhairan B, Hind D, Hutchinson A. Antibiotic prophylaxis for wound infections in total joint arthroplasty: a systematic review. J Bone Joint Surg Br 2008;90(7):915–9.
20. Bratzler DW, Dellinger EP, Olsen KM, et al. Clinical practice guidelines for antimicrobial prophylaxis in

surgery. Surg Infections (Larchmt) 2013;14(1):
73–156.

21. Pachauri A, Acharya KK, Tiwari AK. The effect of tranexamic acid on hemoglobin levels during total
knee arthroplasty. Am J Ther 2014;21(5):366–70.

22. Sarzaeem MM, Razi M, Kazemian G, et al.
Comparing efficacy of three methods of tranexamic
acid administration in reducing hemoglobin drop
following total knee arthroplasty. J Arthroplasty
2014;29(8):1521–4.

23. Tranexamic acid: drug information 2017;156. Available
at: https://www.drugs.com/cdi/tranexamic-acid-tab-
lets.html. Accessed June 20, 2017.

24. Alvarez JC, Santiveri FX, Ramos I, et al. Tranexamic
acid reduces blood transfusion in total knee arthroplasty even when a blood conservation program is
applied. Transfusion 2008;48(3):519–25.

25. Zhang P, Liang Y, He J, et al. Timing of tourniquet
release in total knee arthroplasty: a meta-analysis.
Medicine 2017;96(17):e6786.

26. Olivecrona C, Ponzer S, Hamberg P, et al. Lower
tourniquet cuff pressure reduces postoperative
wound complications after total knee arthroplasty:
a randomized controlled study of 164 patients.
J Bone Joint Surg Am 2012;94(24):2216–21.

27. Fisher WD, Turpie AG. Outpatient thromboprophylaxis after hip or knee surgery: discrepancies and
concerns. CMAJ 2008;178(12):1571–2.

28. Vaishya R, Vijay V, Demesugh DM, et al. Surgical
approaches for total knee arthroplasty. J Clin
Orthop Trauma 2016;7(2):71–9.

29. Weinhardt C, Barisic M, Bergmann EG, et al. Early
results of subvastus versus medial parapatellar
approach in primary total knee arthroplasty. Arch
Orthopaedic Trauma Surg 2004;124(6):401–3.

30. Jung YB, Lee YS, Lee EY, et al. Comparison of the
modified subvastus and medial parapatellar approaches in total knee arthroplasty. Int Orthopaedics 2009;33(2):419–23.

31. Berger RA, Sanders S, Gerlinger T, et al. Outpatient
total knee arthroplasty with a minimally invasive
technique. J Arthroplasty 2005;20(7 Suppl 3):33–8.

32. Cross MB, Berger R. Feasibility and safety of performing outpatient unicompartmental knee arthroplasty. Int Orthopaedics 2014;38(2):443–7.

33. Reilly KA, Beard DJ, Barker KL, et al. Efficacy of an
accelerated recovery protocol for oxford unicompartmental knee arthroplasty–a randomised
controlled trial. The Knee 2005;12(5):351–7.

34. Nguyen LC, Lehil MS, Bozic KJ. Trends in total knee
arthroplasty implant utilization. J Arthroplasty 2015;
30(5):739–42.

35. Beal MD, Delagramaticas D, Fitz D. Improving outcomes in total knee arthroplasty-do navigation or
customized implants have a role? J Orthop Surg
Res 2016;11(1):60.

36. McGrory B, Weber K, Lynott JA, et al. The American academy of orthopaedic surgeons evidence-
based clinical practice guideline on surgical
management of osteoarthritis of the knee. J Bone
Joint Surg Am 2016;98(8):688–92.

37. Haaker RG, Stockheim M, Kamp M, et al. Computer-assisted navigation increases precision of
component placement in total knee arthroplasty.
Clin Orthopaedics Relat Res 2005;(433):152–9.

38. Khakha RS, Chowdhry M, Norris M, et al. Five-year
follow-up of minimally invasive computer assisted
total knee arthroplasty (MICATKA) versus conventional computer assisted total knee arthroplasty
(CATKA) - a population matched study. The Knee
2014;21(5):944–8.

39. Kehlet H, Wilmore DW. Multimodal strategies to
improve surgical outcome. Am J Surg 2002;183(6):
630–41.

40. Berger RA, Kusuma SK, Sanders SA, et al. The feasibility and perioperative complications of outpatient
knee arthroplasty. Clin Orthopaedics Relat Res
2009;467(6):1443–9.

41. Kort NP, Bemelmans YF, van der Kuy PH, et al. Patient selection criteria for outpatient joint arthroplasty. Knee Surg Sports Traumatol Arthrosc 2017;
25(9):2668–75.

42. Ljungqvist O, Scott M, Fearon KC. Enhanced recovery after surgery. JAMA Surg 2017;152(3):292–8.

43. Minns Lowe CJ, Barker KL, Dewey M, et al. Effectiveness of physiotherapy exercise after knee
arthroplasty for osteoarthritis: systematic review
and meta-analysis of randomised controlled trials.
BMJ 2007;335(7624):812.

44. Harvey LA, Brosseau L, Herbert RD. Continuous
passive motion following total knee arthroplasty
in people with arthritis. Cochrane Database Syst
Rev 2014;(2):CD004260.

45. Isaac D, Falode T, Liu P, et al. Accelerated rehabilitation after total knee replacement. The Knee
2005;12(5):346–50.

46. Jones DL, Cauley JA, Kriska AM, et al. Physical activity
and risk of revision total knee arthroplasty in individuals with knee osteoarthritis: a matched case-control
study. J Rheumatol 2004;31(7):1384–90.

47. Ko V, Naylor J, Harris I, et al. One-to-one therapy is
not superior to group or home-based therapy after
total knee arthroplasty: a randomized, superiority
trial. J Bone Joint Surg Am 2013;95(21):1942–9.

Total Hip Arthroplasty in the Outpatient Setting
What You Need to Know (Part 1)

Zain Sayeed, MD, MHA[a], Leila Abaab, MD[a,b],
Mouhanad El-Othmani, MD[a], Vinay Pallekonda, MD[b],
William Mihalko, MD, PhD[c],
Khaled J. Saleh, MD, MSc, FRCS(C), MHCM, CPE[a,*]

KEYWORDS

- Outpatient total joint arthroplasty • Total hip arthroplasty • Length of stay • Early discharge
- Perioperative blood management

KEY POINTS

- The Anesthesiologists Physical Status Classification System and the Charlson Comorbidity Index have often been used as surrogates for arthroplasty selection and risk assessment.
- The components of a given education course may be institution-specific; however, most courses have an underlying theme to empower patients to participate in their recovery and manager their expectations.
- Preoperative patient blood management protocols using epoeitin-alpha may be amenable to reduce length of stay, as they have been associated with reduced transfusion rates in elective total hip arthroplasty.

INTRODUCTION

Total hip arthroplasty (THA) improves quality of life in patients with end-stage osteoarthritis of the hip.[1] The number of primary THA procedures in the United States is projected to rise from 470,000 in 2012 to 700,000 procedures by 2030.[2–4] In preparation for this rise in volume, a concerted effort has been placed upon understanding the value of standardized care pathways in orthopedic surgery.[5] Since the 1990s, there has been a rise in performing hip arthroplasties by various techniques intended to improve recovery and outcome after surgery.[6] Adult reconstruction literature has often coined these protocols with terms such as rapid

recovery, fast-track, and enhanced recovery programs (ERPs).[1,7–9]

Interest in outpatient arthroplasty is also fueled by financial considerations including the ability to minimize costs of an episode of care, physician ownership of ambulatory surgical centers, and the ability for a surgeon to control his or her operating room environment efficiently. Furthermore, outpatient surgical pathways have historically improved patient care and are linked with patient satisfaction.[10–15]

Although outpatient arthroplasty has been recently adopted, it has been successfully implemented throughout the past decade.[10–15] Success is often associated with standardized perioperative protocols, discharge planning,

Funding Sources: No additional funding sources were used for this article.

Conflicts of Interest: No conflicts of interest are evident for authors of this article.

[a] Department of Orthopaedics, Detroit Medical Center, 4201 St Antoine Street, Detroit, MI 48201, USA; [b] Department of Anesthesiology – NorthStar Anesthesia at Detroit Medical Center, 4201 St Antoine Street, Detroit, MI 48201, USA; [c] Campbell Clinic Department of Orthopaedic Surgery & Biomedical Engineering University of Tennessee, 956 Court Avenue, Memphis, TN 32116, USA

* Corresponding author.

E-mail address: kjsaleh@gmail.com

multidisciplinary coordination, and rehabilitation planning. Previous studies have found that outpatient THA pathways are safe, effective, and do not increase incidence of peri- and postoperative complications.[10–15]

This article will discuss all components involved in creating and implementing a successful outpatient THA pathway. Specifically, reviews patient selection criteria, preoperative education, and preoperative medical optimization.

PREOPERATIVE CONSIDERATIONS FOR OUTPATIENT TOTAL HIP ARTHROPLASTY
Patient Selection Criteria

The Anesthesiologists Physical Status Classification System (ASA-PS) and the Charlson Comorbidity Index (CCI) have often been used as surrogates for arthroplasty selection and risk assessment. Although these measures are accepted in the general medical community, they were not developed with the intent to safely select outpatient THA candidates. With the inevitable demand for hip arthroplasty in the outpatient setting, specific and predictive medical risk stratification has become necessary to allow patients to receive value-based care without subjecting the patient to potential rush surgeries. The following section will discuss existing risk stratification tools, then delves into orthopedic-specific tools recently developed by arthroplasty specialists for consideration of outpatient THA.

The ASA-PS score is often used in preoperative settings as a medical screening tool for arthroplasty procedures.[16,17] The ASA-PS score consists of 6 classification groups with numerically worsening physical status:

1. A generally healthy person
2. A patient with some systemic diseases
3. A patient with severe systemic disease
4. A patient with a systemic disease that is a constant threat to life
5. A moribund patient who is not expected to survive without the planned surgery

Although the ASA-PS classification is a validated risk stratification measure, there have been reports of interobserver variability in assignment of ASA-PS scores to patients.[18,19] Notably, the ASA-PS classification was not designed to assess operative risk; rather it was designed to stratify physical status before selecting appropriate anesthesia regimens for surgery. Operative risk is a broader consideration including not only physical status, but also the nature of the procedure and other factors like preoperative

optimization and preventative postoperative management. Even if the ASA-PS was a valid measure of operative risk, ordinal classifications limit precision and selection for outpatient THA. Furthermore, ASA-PS has not been validated in rapid recovery THA programs, and is not predictive for early discharge.

The CCI was developed to offer a general prediction of 1-year mortality by utilization of medical chart data.[20] Primarily designed to be used in clinical studies and research methodology, the CCI consisted of 19 comorbidities, each assigned a weight from 1, for conditions such as congestive heart failure, to 6, for metastatic solid tumors or acquired immune deficiency syndrome. The CCI was a sum of its weighted scores. Currently, the CCI has been adjusted to be used in conjunction with administrative health care codes such as the International Classification of Disease (ICD) system.[21–23] More often than not, the CCI does not measure all comorbidities relevant to arthroplasty procedures, and does not account for severity of comorbidities. Different versions of the CCI have demonstrated validity in certain populations, but results are largely dependent on study design and outcomes of interest. Thus, although argued to be useful in research settings, the CCI does not address safe selection criteria for outpatient THA patients.

Literature is lacking with regard to arthroplasty-specific guidelines for outpatient THA selection; however, some evidence associates pre-existing conditions with adverse events (AEs) after outpatient arthroplasty. In a clinical review by Kort and colleagues,[24] researchers stressed the important patient inclusion and exclusion criteria for outpatient arthroplasty. Currently, there remains a lack of randomized controlled trials (RCTs) assessing patient selection criteria for outpatient arthroplasty procedures. Most studies assessing outpatient THA report outcomes on preselected patients.[6,15,25–27] The ability and willingness of a patient to participate in an outpatient procedure often dictates the primary benchmark of inclusion.[6,15,25–27] Most studies identified utilization of ASA-PS classification for patients as an added inclusion criteria.[6,15,25–27] ASA-PS scores of greater than 2 and bleeding disorders were associated with AEs (revision, infection, mortality, deep venous thrombosis [DVT], and wound complications).[28] Patients were generally operated if they were younger than 65, with age ranges of 45 to 80 years.[12,15,26] Outpatient arthroplasty literature suggests that older age (>75 years) is a risk factor for postoperative falls, pain, urinary retention, and higher risk for readmission within 1 year.

Patients older than 80 years of age demonstrated the highest risk of falls and readmissions.[29]

Preoperative cardiac clearance was recommended if patients had a history of cardiovascular risk.[6,15,25–27] In all studies, patients with heart failure were at higher risk for readmission, and patients with severe cardiac comorbidities alongside an ASA-PS score greater than 2 were not included for outpatient arthroplasty.[6,15,25–27] Dorr and colleagues[26] identified postoperative hypotension as a clinical factor associated with delayed discharge. Furthermore, 1 study identified difficulties associated with coordinating home discharge as an etiology for delay.[26] Particularly, researchers did not reveal why patients were not discharged home; however, the fear of early discharge without postoperative dependence on someone else may have led to delayed discharge. A study by Callaghan and colleagues[28] demonstrated dependent functional status (partial or total) was associated with increased readmission with outpatient THA. Therefore, both preoperative screening and preparing the home environment for disposition are necessary components for preventing prolonged discharge in outpatient THA.[6,15,25–27]

Just as inclusion criteria are necessary for successful implementation of outpatient arthroplasty pathways, it is also imperative to establish stringent exclusion criteria. Most studies excluded patients with cardiac (history of myocardial infarction, arrhythmia, and heart failure) and pulmonary (respiratory failure) comorbidities.[6,15,25–27] One study excluded patients with diabetes mellitus (DM) type 1 and 2. Additionally, body mass index (BMI) has been associated studied as a risk factor in outpatient arthroplasty.[15,30,31] Berger and colleagues[13] excluded patients with a high BMI (>40 m²/kg). Ibrahim and colleagues further supported Berger and colleagues outpatient pathway by associating high BMI (>40 m²/kg) with increased operative time and intraoperative blood loss in THA.[29] Researchers extended their correlation by describing increased technical difficulties associated with obese patients.[29] On the contrary, Husted and colleagues reported a lack of correlation between prolonged hospital stay and BMI in their outpatient THA cohort.[28] The authors conclude that a high BMI (>30 m²/kg) may warrant as a cautionary or general exclusion criteria for outpatient THA.

Perhaps one of the more prevalent conditions of patients undergoing joint arthroplasty is chronic renal disease (CRD).[32] Warth and colleagues[32] suggest patients with CRD are at greater risk for AEs. Patients with stage 3 to 5 CRD were at a twofold increased risk for mortality following THA.[32] The authors recommend preoperative screening for renal function in patients considered as candidates for outpatient THA. They also recommend patients with moderate-to-severe CRD or renal impairment be excluded from outpatient care pathways for possibility of an extended postoperative course.

Another risk factor to consider for outpatient THA patients includes opioid consumption. Pivec and colleagues[33] assessed 54 patients who had required opioid analgesia 3 months prior to THA with a matched cohort of opioid-naïve patients. Patients who used narcotics prior to THA were likely to suffer from opioid-induced hyperalgesia and demonstrated a prolonged hospital stay.[33] Because of higher management burden of analgesia treatment, Kort and colleagues[24] suggested the exclusion of outpatient THA patients with a history of opioid analgesia.

In efforts to safely select patients for outpatient THA while considering both risk stratification scoring and exclusion criteria, Meneghini and colleagues[34] described use of an outpatient arthroplasty risk assessment (OARA) score. The OARA score was developed by an adult reconstruction specialist alongside an internal medicine physician, both with over a decade of experience in ERPs for total joint arthroplasty (TJA) patients. The OARA score assessed 9 comorbidity categories scored upon presence, severity, medical optimization, and control of the listed conditions.[34] The categorizations included general medical, hematologic, cardiac, endocrine, gastrointestinal, neurologic/psychological, renal, pulmonary, and infectious disease-related comorbid conditions.[34] The positive predictive value (PPV) of the OARA score to identify outpatient TJA candidates compared with CCI and ASA-PS scores proved to be robust and appropriate for outpatient or short-stay TJA patients.[34] Although the study was limited in describing how to derive the OARA score, the PPV for OARA score was 81.6% for the same- or next-day discharge, compared with 56.4 for ASA-PS scores ($P<.001$) and 70.3 for CCI scores ($P = .002$).[34] A summary of the authors' general inclusion criteria is available in Table 1.

OPTIMIZING PATIENTS FOR OUTPATIENT TOTAL HIP ARTHROPLASTY
Preoperative Education Programs for Outpatient Total Hip Arthroplasty
Preoperative education programs for patients undergoing outpatient THA have been reported to enhance ERPs. The components of a given education course may be institution-specific;

Table 1
General inclusion and exclusion criteria for outpatient total hip arthroplasty

Inclusion Criteria	Exclusion Criteria
• Age <75 y • ASA < III • Determined discharge destination	• Bleeding disorders • Poorly controlled cardiac conditions (eg, heart failure, arrhythmia) • History of pulmonary embolism • History of respiratory failure • Uncontrolled diabetes mellitus (type 1 or 2) • BMI >30 m²/kg • Chronic opioid consumption • Functional neurologic impairments • Chronic/end-stage renal disease

however, most courses have an underlying theme to empower patients to participate in their recovery and manage their expectations.[35] Some studies have shown a correlation between preoperative education and patient-reported outcome measures (PROMs), such as satisfaction.[36–38] Yoon and colleagues[35] prospectively examined 261 patients undergoing primary unilateral TJAs paired with a one-on-one education program. Researchers reported a reduced length of stay (LOS) by approximately 1 day than nonparticipants for both total hip and total knee arthroplasty.[35] Preoperative education has also been estimated to reduce costs.[39]

An RCT by Giraudet-Le Quintrec and colleagues[40] assessed the positive effect of patient education for hip surgery. The study prospectively evaluated patients scheduled for elective primary THA. Patients were randomly assigned into 2 groups. Group 1 attended a preoperative multidisciplinary information session 2 to 6 weeks prior to surgery, whereas the control group did not. All patients completed a state anxiety inventory (SAI) before surgery and then 1 and 7 days after surgery.[40] Patients who attended the informative sessions with routine verbal information found a preoperative reduction in anxiety and pain compared with those receiving the briefing.[40] Therefore, the authors recommend live in-person arthroplasty class prior to surgical intervention for outpatient candidates.

Blood Management in Outpatient Total Hip Arthroplasty

Perioperative anemia is a common complication found in arthroplasty procedures, concerning approximately 15% to 25% of patients preoperatively, and nearly 80% of patients postoperatively.[41,42] Hip arthroplasty literature demonstrates that preoperative anemia increases the incidence of intraoperative and postoperative morbidity and mortality.[43] Several studies utilizing retrospective data have shown that preoperative patient blood management (PBM) protocols using epoeitin-alpha (EPO), were able to reduce transfusion in elective THA.[44] Additionally, other studies have demonstrated adjuvant intravenous tranexamic acid or iron therapy in the pre-, intra-, or postoperative setting may decrease rates of transfusion.[45,46] The presentation of the anemic orthopedic patient is variable, and a given surgeon must rely upon hematological indices. Postoperative transfusion is generally reserved for patients who are symptomatic and also have Hb levels of less than 8 g/dL. Additionally, symptomatic patients with higher Hb levels may also require transfusion.

In a quality improvement project reported by Dwyer and colleagues,[47] an ERP was implemented to optimize hospital stay following THA. The study compared a group of 64 ERP patients with a historic cohort of 63 patients who received conventional care. Researchers reported that 1 factor linked with earlier discharge was an Hb level of greater than 14 g/dL at the time of surgery.[47] The correction of Hb levels to greater than 12 g/dL preoperatively has been associated with reduced need for transfusion in the postoperative setting and earlier discharge.[48]

Generally, treatment protocols for anemic arthroplasty patients follow a specific regimen:

> EPO and/or oral or intravenous iron in the preoperative period
> Tranexamic acid in pre-, intra- or postoperative phases
> Iron after surgery

In a recent study by Rineau and colleagues,[49] patients were given a PBM protocol if their Hb in their preoperative visit was less than 13 g/dL. In this case, intravenous ferrous carboxymaltose was administered alongside the first EPO injection 4 weeks prior to operation. In the intra- and postoperative periods, tranexamic acid was used systematically in absence of contraindication, and FCM was recommended for postoperative anemic patients. A restrictive single-unit transfusion strategy was endorsed with Hb readings ranging from 7 to 8 g/dL as transfusion triggers; however, higher triggers were used pending patient comorbidities. Three hundred sixty-seven patients were assessed, and researchers reported a significant decrease in transfusion rate and number of patients with Hb level of less than 10 g/dL at time of discharge.

The correction of anemia prior to THA surgery has been associated with reduced surgical risk, hospital cost, and shorter stay.[50] The use of oral iron therapy has been studied and is frequently used in many preoperative regimens for anemic patients. Although some studies have shown that oral iron therapy may reduce the incidence of anemia prior to joint replacement,[50] the clinical value of iron supplementation postoperatively has been debated.[51] Currently, no consensus or practice guideline exits in the orthopedic literature that summarizes a methodology to treat anemia with oral iron therapy.

Utilization of tranexamic acid (TXA) to minimize perioperative blood loss associated with THA has been extensively studied.[52,53] TXA is a synthetic pharmacologic agent that limits blood loss by inhibiting fibrinolysis. Specifically, TXA reversibly binds and saturates lysine sites of plasminogen, thus preventing its activation to plasmin. This inhibits the degradation of fibrin, as plasmin is designed to bind to the surface of fibrin in order to initiate breakdown of a clot. TXA is available in several forms: intravenous, topical, and oral. Lee and colleagues[54] have assessed the utilization of oral TXA in primary hip arthroplasty. In their study, 54 patients received a 1 or 2 g oral dose of TXA preoperatively, and at 6 and 12 hours postoperatively. The trial cohort was compared with a matched control group of 54 patients who did not receive any form of TXA for their primary THA. Lee and colleagues reported higher postoperative hemoglobin (10.3 vs 9.4 g/dL), lower hemoglobin drop (3.0 vs 4.1 g/dL) and hidden blood loss (149 vs 354 mL), and lower actual total blood loss (847 vs 1096 mL). The researchers concluded that oral TXA is a feasible option to reduce blood loss in primary THA.

Typically doses for intravenous TXA administration in TJA are 1 to 2 g in the perioperative setting. In many published studies, the use of intravenous TXA in THA ranges from 10 to 20 mg/kg, and several studies report a standard 1g dose. Other studies have used a TXA bolus preoperatively, followed by intraoperative infusion.[55] Contraindications for TXA include previous history of allergy/hypersensitivity, active thromboembolic disease, and seizure disorder.[56–63] TXA is able to cross the blood barrier and has potential to induce seizures due to glycine receptor interaction.[56–63] TXA is renally

cleared from the body; therefore adjustments should be made in patients with compromised renal function, but this does not subdue its application. With regard to potential complications associated with TXA in TJA, studies often focus on venous thromboembolic (VTE) events. Meta-analyses report no increased risk of VTE after use of TXA for TJA.[56–63] Whether a patient is able to receive outpatient TJA without TXA administration has not been fully elucidated in the orthopedic literature.

Medical Management

Hypertension is one of the most prevalent diseases among patients undergoing primary THA,[64] and heightened focus should be allocated to its management in the perioperative period, as it constitutes a substantial risk factor for postoperative myocardial infarction (MI).[65,66] Some antihypertensive medications, such as diuretics, ACEIs, and ARBs, should be stopped 24 to 48 hours preoperatively, as they may interfere with hemodynamics and electrolyte balance.[67] Some other classes of hypertension medications, such as beta-blockers, should not be interrupted, and should be given perioperatively.[68,69] As soon as an oral route is permitted and hemodynamics are stable, the authors recommend resuming hypertension medications to avoid any complications.

MI is a feared complication in patients with coronary artery disease undergoing primary THA, as coronary history is correlated with long-term mortality following THA.[70] Having a stent does not protect against postoperative MI. Kumar and colleagues[71] reported that patients with stent and a history of MI had the highest risk for postoperative MI, and elective joint replacement should be postponed at least 1 year after a cardiac event or stent placement. Intraoperative stability of hemodynamics should be observed, and any hypotension should be avoided. Systematic troponin testing in the postoperative setting has been suggested by Bass and colleagues,[72] who reported that approximately 13% of subclinical MI had been diagnosed in high-risk patients after THA.

Thromboembolic diseases and especially deep venous thrombosis (DVT) are common in TJA patients.[73,74] Zhang and colleagues[75] identified past history of DVT, varicose veins, and CHF as major risk factors associated with DVT following primary THA. Other risk factors were female gender, age (≥80), hypertension, (active) cancer, obesity (BMI≥30), and (black) race. Notably, patients undergoing primary THA have a decreased risk of AEs when regional anesthesia is implemented compared with general anesthesia.[76] Therefore, the authors recommend regional anesthesia whenever possible. In order to prevent these complications, chemical prophylaxis with low-molecular-weight heparin LMWH, fondaparinux, or adjusted-dose vitamin K antagonist (international normalized ratio [INR] target, 2.5; range, 2.0–3.0) for 28 to 35 days has been suggested in patients primary THA.[77] Aspirin may also be considered for postoperative thromboprophylaxis in the outpatient THA setting. Early mobilization is also recommended after THA.[78,79] In the setting of outpatient THA, Colwell described a newer portable device that allows compression at home while the patient is ambulating.[73] Rehabilitation protocols for outpatient THA will be reviewed in later sections.

Diabetes mellitus is another common pathology encountered in patients undergoing THA. Studies have linked this comorbidity with surgical site infections and postoperative wound complications among other complications.[80] Han and colleagues[81] reported that poorly controlled preoperative diabetes (HbA1c $\geq$ 8%) was associated with an increased incidence of postoperative wound complications after TKA. Similarly, Capozzi and colleagues[82] recommended routine screening of all patients undergoing elective THA by systematically having their HbA1c checked. If the latter is increased, surgery should be postponed and patients referred for diabetic counseling.

Renal dysfunction is also associated with longer hospital stay and higher mortality,[83,84] which makes renal function optimization a paramount. All medications used perioperatively such as narcotics, muscle relaxants, NSAIDs, and antibiotics should be adapted to the renal function. Close monitoring of serum creatinine following joint arthroplasty is also recommended.[85]

SUMMARY

Part 1 of this series discussed components involved in creating and implementing a successful outpatient THA pathway. Specifically, it reviewed patient selection criteria, preoperative education, and preoperative medical optimization. Each of these components aids in creation of a streamlined method by which THA patients will receive high-value care. Although, there is no gold standard for preoperative optimization of outpatient THA patients, evidence-based approaches will likely minimize AEs and improve care nationally (Box 1).

Box 1
General preoperative recommendations for outpatient total hip arthroplasty

- Create patient selection criteria for outptatient THA pathways that is institution-specific
- Medically optimize patients prior to inducting into outpatient THA pathway
- Utilize preoperative blood management protocols for anemic patients
- Utilize preferred method of TXA administration depending on institution review of evidenced-based recommendations
- Enhance patient activation by creating live joint classes and workshops to reduce patient anxiety and answer possible patient inquiry

REFERENCES

1. Ethgen O, Bruyere O, Richy F, et al. Health-related quality of life in total hip and total knee arthroplasty. A qualitative and systematic review of the literature. J Bone Joint Surg Am 2004;86-A(5): 963–74.
2. Kurtz S, Ong K, Lau E, et al. Projections of primary and revision hip and knee arthroplasty in the United States from 2005 to 2030. J Bone Joint Surg Am 2007;89(4):780–5.
3. Kurtz SM, Ong KL, Lau E, et al. Impact of the economic downturn on total joint replacement demand in the United States: updated projections to 2021. J Bone Joint Surg Am 2014;96(8):624–30.
4. Lehil MS, Bozic KJ. Trends in total hip arthroplasty implant utilization in the United States. J Arthroplasty 2014;29(10):1915–8.
5. Saleh KJ, Shaffer WO. Understanding value-based reimbursement models and trends in orthopaedic health policy: an introduction to the Medicare Access and CHIP Reauthorization Act (MACRA) of 2015. J Am Acad Orthop Surg 2016;24(11):e136–47.
6. Aynardi M, Post Z, Ong A, et al. Outpatient surgery as a means of cost reduction in total hip arthroplasty: a case-control study. HSS J 2014;10(3): 252–5.
7. Kim NR, Moon SG, Park JY, et al. Stress ultrasound in baseball players with ulnar collateral ligament injuries: additional value for predicting rehabilitation outcome. J Shoulder Elbow Surg 2017;26(5): 815–23.
8. Pozzi F, Madara K, Zeni JA Jr. A six-week supervised exercise and educational intervention after total hip arthroplasty: a case series. Int J Sports Phys Ther 2017;12(2):259–72.

9. Xu R, Carty MJ, Orgill DP, et al. The teaming curve: a longitudinal study of the influence of surgical team familiarity on operative time. Ann Surg 2013;258(6):953–7.

10. Husted H, Lunn TH, Troelsen A, et al. Why still in hospital after fast-track hip and knee arthroplasty? Acta Orthop 2011;82(6):679–84.

11. Molko S, Combalia A. Rapid recovery programmes for hip and knee arthroplasty. An update. Rev Esp Cir Ortop Traumatol 2017;61(2):130–8.

12. Berger RA, Kusuma SK, Sanders SA, et al. The feasibility and perioperative complications of outpatient knee arthroplasty. Clin Orthop Relat Res 2009; 467(6):1443–9.

13. Berger RA, Sanders S, D'Ambrogio E, et al. Minimally invasive quadriceps-sparing TKA: results of a comprehensive pathway for outpatient TKA. J Knee Surg 2006;19(2):145–8.

14. Berger RA, Sanders S, Gerlinger T, et al. Outpatient total knee arthroplasty with a minimally invasive technique. J Arthroplasty 2005;20(7 Suppl 3): 33–8.

15. Berger RA, Sanders SA, Thill ES, et al. Newer anesthesia and rehabilitation protocols enable outpatient hip replacement in selected patients. Clin Orthop Relat Res 2009;467(6):1424–30.

16. Hackett NJ, De Oliveira GS, Jain UK, et al. ASA class is a reliable independent predictor of medical complications and mortality following surgery. Int J Surg 2015;18:184–90.

17. Schaeffer JF, Scott DJ, Godin JA, et al. The Association of ASA class on total knee and total hip arthroplasty readmission rates in an Academic Hospital. J Arthroplasty 2015;30(5):723–7.

18. Fitz-Henry J. The ASA classification and perioperative risk. Ann R Coll Surg Engl 2011;93(3): 185–7.

19. Mak PH, Campbell RC, Irwin MG. The ASA physical status classification: inter-observer consistency. American Society of Anesthesiologists. Anaesth Intensive Care 2002;30(5):633–40.

20. Charlson ME, Pompei P, Ales KL, et al. A new method of classifying prognostic comorbidity in longitudinal studies: development and validation. J Chronic Dis 1987;40(5):373–83.

21. Romano PS, Roos LL, Jollis JG. Adapting a clinical comorbidity index for use with ICD-9-CM administrative data: differing perspectives. J Clin Epidemiol 1993;46(10):1075–9 [discussion: 1081–90].

22. D'Hoore W, Bouckaert A, Tilquin C. Practical considerations on the use of the Charlson comorbidity index with administrative data bases. J Clin Epidemiol 1996;49(12):1429–33.

23. Ghali WA, Hall RE, Rosen AK, et al. Searching for an improved clinical comorbidity index for use with ICD-9-CM administrative data. J Clin Epidemiol 1996;49(3):273–8.

24. Kort NP, Bemelmans YF, van der Kuy PH, et al. Patient selection criteria for outpatient joint arthroplasty. Knee Surg Sports Traumatol Arthrosc 2017;(25):2668–75.

25. Chen D, Berger RA. Outpatient minimally invasive total hip arthroplasty via a modified Watson-Jones approach: technique and results. Instr Course Lect 2013;62:229–36.

26. Dorr LD, Thomas DJ, Zhu J, et al. Outpatient total hip arthroplasty. J Arthroplasty 2010;25(4):501–6.

27. Hartog YM, Mathijssen NM, Vehmeijer SB. Total hip arthroplasty in an outpatient setting in 27 selected patients. Acta Orthop 2015;86(6):667–70.

28. Callaghan JJ, Pugely A, Liu S, et al. Measuring rapid recovery program outcomes: are all patients candidates for rapid recovery. J Arthroplasty 2015;30(4):531–2.

29. Lovald ST, Ong KL, Lau EC, et al. Patient selection in short stay total hip arthroplasty for medicare patients. J Arthroplasty 2015;30(12):2086–91.

30. Husted H, Holm G, Jacobsen S. Predictors of length of stay and patient satisfaction after hip and knee replacement surgery: fast-track experience in 712 patients. Acta Orthop 2008;79(2):168–73.

31. Ibrahim MS, Khan MA, Nizam I, et al. Peri-operative interventions producing better functional outcomes and enhanced recovery following total hip and knee arthroplasty: an evidence-based review. BMC Med 2013;11:37.

32. Warth LC, Pugely AJ, Martin CT, et al. Total Joint arthroplasty in patients with chronic renal disease: is it worth the risk? J Arthroplasty 2015;30(9 Suppl):51–4.

33. Pivec R, Issa K, Naziri Q, et al. Opioid use prior to total hip arthroplasty leads to worse clinical outcomes. Int orthopaedics 2014;38(6):1159–65.

34. Meneghini RM, Ziemba-Davis M, Ishmael MK, et al. Safe Selection of outpatient joint arthroplasty patients with medical risk stratification: the "outpatient arthroplasty risk assessment score". J Arthroplasty 2017;32(8):2325–31.

35. Yoon RS, Nellans KW, Geller JA, et al. Patient education before hip or knee arthroplasty lowers length of stay. J Arthroplasty 2010;25(4):547–51.

36. Argenson JN, Husted H, Lombardi A Jr, et al. Global forum: An international perspective on outpatient surgical procedures for adult hip and knee reconstruction. J Bone Joint Surg Am 2016; 98(13):e55.

37. Lin PC, Lin LC, Lin JJ. Comparing the effectiveness of different educational programs for patients with total knee arthroplasty. Orthop Nurs 1997;16(5): 43–9.

38. Raphael M, Jaeger M, van Vlymen J. Easily adoptable total joint arthroplasty program allows discharge home in two days. Can J Anaesth 2011; 58(10):902–10.

39. Bierbaum BE, Callaghan JJ, Galante JO, et al. An analysis of blood management in patients having a total hip or knee arthroplasty. J Bone Joint Surg Am 1999;81(1):2–10.

40. Giraudet-Le Quintrec JS, Coste J, Vastel L, et al. Positive effect of patient education for hip surgery: a randomized trial. Clin Orthop Relat Res 2003;(414):112–20.

41. Spahn DR. Anemia and patient blood management in hip and knee surgery: a systematic review of the literature. Anesthesiology 2010;113(2):482–95.

42. Lasocki S, Krauspe R, von Heymann C, et al. PRE-PARE: the prevalence of perioperative anaemia and need for patient blood management in elective orthopaedic surgery: a multicentre, observational study. Eur J Anaesthesiol 2015;32(3):160–7.

43. Myers E, O'Grady P, Dolan AM. The influence of preclinical anaemia on outcome following total hip replacement. Arch Orthop Trauma Surg 2004;124(10):699–701.

44. Kotze A, Carter LA, Scally AJ. Effect of a patient blood management programme on preoperative anaemia, transfusion rate, and outcome after primary hip or knee arthroplasty: a quality improvement cycle. Br J Anaesth 2012;108(6):943–52.

45. Ker K, Edwards P, Perel P, et al. Effect of tranexamic acid on surgical bleeding: systematic review and cumulative meta-analysis. BMJ 2012;344:e3054.

46. Ker K, Prieto-Merino D, Roberts I. Systematic review, meta-analysis and meta-regression of the effect of tranexamic acid on surgical blood loss. Br J Surg 2013;100(10):1271–9.

47. Dwyer AJ, Tarassoli P, Thomas W, et al. Enhanced recovery program in total hip arthroplasty. Indian J Orthop 2012;46(4):407–12.

48. Rogers BA, Cowie A, Alcock C, et al. Identification and treatment of anaemia in patients awaiting hip replacement. Ann R Coll Surg Engl 2008;90(6):504–7.

49. Rineau E, Chaudet A, Chassier C, et al. Implementing a blood management protocol during the entire perioperative period allows a reduction in transfusion rate in major orthopedic surgery: a before-after study. Transfusion 2016;56(3):673–81.

50. Andrews CM, Lane DW, Bradley JG. Iron pre-load for major joint replacement. Transfus Med 1997;7(4):281–6.

51. Mundy GM, Birtwistle SJ, Power RA. The effect of iron supplementation on the level of haemoglobin after lower limb arthroplasty. J Bone Joint Surg Br 2005;87(2):213–7.

52. Niskanen RO, Korkala OL. Tranexamic acid reduces blood loss in cemented hip arthroplasty: a randomized, double-blind study of 39 patients with osteoarthritis. Acta Orthop 2005;76(6):829–32.

53. Zhou XD, Tao LJ, Li J, et al. Do we really need tranexamic acid in total hip arthroplasty? A meta-analysis of nineteen randomized controlled trials. Arch Orthop Trauma Surg 2013;133(7):1017–27.

54. Lee QJ, Chang WY, Wong YC. Blood-sparing efficacy of oral tranexamic acid in primary total hip arthroplasty. J Arthroplasty 2017;32(1):139–42.

55. Lemay E, Guay J, Cote C, et al. Tranexamic acid reduces the need for allogenic red blood cell transfusions in patients undergoing total hip replacement. Can J Anaesth 2004;51(1):31–7.

56. Evangelista PJ, Aversano MW, Koli E, et al. Effect of tranexamic acid on transfusion rates following total joint arthroplasty: a cost and comparative effectiveness analysis. Orthop Clin North Am 2017;48(2):109–15.

57. Kayupov E, Fillingham YA, Okroj K, et al. Oral and intravenous tranexamic acid are equivalent at reducing blood loss following total hip arthroplasty: a randomized controlled trial. J Bone Joint Surg Am 2017;99(5):373–8.

58. Li JF, Li H, Zhao H, et al. Combined use of intravenous and topical versus intravenous tranexamic acid in primary total knee and hip arthroplasty: a meta-analysis of randomised controlled trials. J Orthop Surg Res 2017;12(1):22.

59. Liu X, Liu J, Sun G. A comparison of combined intravenous and topical administration of tranexamic acid with intravenous tranexamic acid alone for blood loss reduction after total hip arthroplasty: a meta-analysis. Int J Surg 2017;41:34–43.

60. Ollivier JE, Van Driessche S, Billuart F, et al. Tranexamic acid and total hip arthroplasty: optimizing the administration method. Ann Transl Med 2016;4(24):530.

61. Sabbag OD, Abdel MP, Amundson AW, et al. Tranexamic acid was safe in arthroplasty patients with a history of venous thromboembolism: a matched outcome study. J Arthroplasty 2017;32(9S):S246–50.

62. Xie J, Hu Q, Huang Q, et al. Comparison of intravenous versus topical tranexamic acid in primary total hip and knee arthroplasty: An updated meta-analysis. Thromb Res 2017;153:28–36.

63. Zhang H, He G, Zhang C, et al. Is combined topical and intravenous tranexamic acid superior to intravenous tranexamic acid alone for controlling blood loss after total hip arthroplasty?: a meta-analysis. Medicine 2017;96(21):e6916.

64. Piano LP, Golmia RP, Scheinberg M. Total hip and knee joint replacement: perioperative clinical aspects. Einstein (Sao Paulo) 2010;8(3):350–3.

65. Dy CJ, Wilkinson JD, Tamariz L, et al. Influence of preoperative cardiovascular risk factor clusters on complications of total joint arthroplasty. Am J Orthop (Belle Mead NJ) 2011;40(11):560–5.

66. Belmont PJ Jr, Goodman GP, Kusnezov NA, et al. Postoperative myocardial infarction and cardiac arrest following primary total knee and hip

arthroplasty: rates, risk factors, and time of occurrence. J Bone Joint Surg Am 2014;96(24):2025–31.

67. Calloway JJ, Memtsoudis SG, Krauser DG, et al. Hemodynamic effects of angiotensin inhibitors in elderly hypertensives undergoing total knee arthroplasty under regional anesthesia. J Am Soc Hypertens 2014;8(9):644–51.

68. Blessberger H, Kammler J, Steinwender C. Perioperative use of beta-blockers in cardiac and noncardiac surgery. JAMA 2015;313(20):2070–1.

69. Varon J, Marik PE. Perioperative hypertension management. Vasc Health Risk Manag 2008;4(3):615–27.

70. Gaston MS, Amin AK, Clayton RA, et al. Does a history of cardiac disease or hypertension increase mortality following primary elective total hip arthroplasty? Surgeon 2007;5(5):260–5.

71. Kumar A, Tsai WC, Tan TS, et al. Risk of Post-TKA acute myocardial infarction in patients with a history of myocardial infarction or coronary stent. Clin Orthop Relat Res 2016;474(2):479–86.

72. Bass AR, Rodriguez T, Hyun G, et al. Myocardial ischaemia after hip and knee arthroplasty: incidence and risk factors. Int orthopaedics 2015;39(10):2011–6.

73. Colwell CW Jr. What is the state of the art in orthopaedic thromboprophylaxis in lower extremity reconstruction? Instr Course Lect 2011;60:283–90.

74. Rahme E, Dasgupta K, Burman M, et al. Postdischarge thromboprophylaxis and mortality risk after hip-or knee-replacement surgery. CMAJ 2008;178(12):1545–54.

75. Zhang J, Chen Z, Zheng J, et al. Risk factors for venous thromboembolism after total hip and total knee arthroplasty: a meta-analysis. Arch Orthop Trauma Surg 2015;135(6):759–72.

76. Roderick P, Ferris G, Wilson K, et al. Towards evidence-based guidelines for the prevention of venous thromboembolism: systematic reviews of mechanical methods, oral anticoagulation, dextran and regional anaesthesia as thromboprophylaxis. Health Technol Assess 2005;9(49):iii–iv [ix-x, 1–78].

77. Geerts WH, Pineo GF, Heit JA, et al. Prevention of venous thromboembolism: the Seventh ACCP Conference on Antithrombotic and Thrombolytic Therapy. Chest 2004;126(3 Suppl):338s–400s.

78. Husted H, Otte KS, Kristensen BB, et al. Low risk of thromboembolic complications after fast-track hip and knee arthroplasty. Acta Orthop 2010;81(5):599–605.

79. Chandrasekaran S, Ariaretnam SK, Tsung J, et al. Early mobilization after total knee replacement reduces the incidence of deep venous thrombosis. ANZ J Surg 2009;79(7–8):526–9.

80. Moon HK, Han CD, Yang IH, et al. Factors affecting outcome after total knee arthroplasty in patients with diabetes mellitus. Yonsei Med J 2008;49(1):129–37.

81. Han HS, Kang SB. Relations between long-term glycemic control and postoperative wound and infectious complications after total knee arthroplasty in type 2 diabetics. Clin Orthop Surg 2013;5(2):118–23.

82. Capozzi JD, Lepkowsky ER, Callari MM, et al. The prevalence of diabetes mellitus and routine hemoglobin a1c screening in elective total joint arthroplasty patients. J Arthroplasty 2017;32(1):304–8.

83. Nielson E, Hennrikus E, Lehman E, et al. Angiotensin axis blockade, hypotension, and acute kidney injury in elective major orthopedic surgery. J Hosp Med 2014;9(5):283–8.

84. Jafari SM, Huang R, Joshi A, et al. Renal impairment following total joint arthroplasty: who is at risk? J Arthroplasty 2010;25(6 Suppl):49–53, 53.e1–2.

85. Aeng ES, Shalansky KF, Lau TT, et al. Acute kidney injury with tobramycin-impregnated bone cement spacers in prosthetic joint infections. Ann Pharmacother 2015;49(11):1207–13.

Total Hip Arthroplasty in the Outpatient Setting
What You Need to Know (Part 2)

Zain Sayeed, MD, MHA[a], Leila Abaab, MD[a,b],
Mouhanad El-Othmani, MD[a], Vinay Pallekonda, MD[b],
William Mihalko, MD, PhD[c],
Khaled J. Saleh, MD, MSc, FRCS(C), MHCM, CPE[a,*]

KEYWORDS

- Outpatient total joint arthroplasty • Total hip arthroplasty • Length of stay • Early discharge
- Spinal anesthesia • Rehabilitation

KEY POINTS

- General anesthesia is known to be associated with postoperative drowsiness and hypotension that might interfere with the fast-track protocols. General anesthesia, if used, will be done with sevoflurane and fentanyl in addition to peripheral nerve blocks.
- Intraoperative room efficiency may be optimized by minimizing staff turnover, traffic flow, and the size of the surgical team.
- Regional anesthesia allows for less narcotic administration, which has been associated with decreased postoperative nausea and hypotension.

INTRODUCTION

Outpatient total hip arthroplasty (THA) has become increasingly adopted by orthopedic surgeons and hospital systems across the nation. Over the past decade, orthopedic literature has trended toward reporting outpatient arthroplasty outcomes associated with enhanced recovery pathways (ERPs).[1–6] Most outpatient THA studies often correlate higher-value care with standardized care pathways, improved discharge planning, minimally invasive techniques, and fast-track rehabilitation. Outpatient THA pathways have been reported as cost-effective and do not increase risk of peri- and postoperative complications.[1–6]

This article is the second installment of understanding the components involved in creating and implementing a successful outpatient THA pathway. This article reviews intraoperative factors involved in outpatient THA such as anesthesia and analgesia modalities, operative techniques, and intraoperative efficiency. Finally, it elaborates on postoperative considerations for outpatient THA including rehabilitation.

ANESTHESIA AND ANALGESIA MODALITIES

With growing emphasis on cost efficiency, optimizing anesthesia protocols has become essential to assure rapid rehabilitation and enable a minimally invasive outpatient approach to THA.

General Anesthesia

General anesthesia is known to be associated with postoperative drowsiness and hypotension

---

Funding Sources: No additional funding sources were used for this article.
Conflicts of Interest: No conflicts of interest are evident for authors of this article.
[a] Department of Orthopaedics, Detroit Medical Center, 4201 St Antoine Street, Detroit, MI 48201, USA; [b] Department of Anesthesiology – NorthStar Anesthesia at Detroit Medical Center, 4201 St Antoine Street, Detroit, MI 48201, USA; [c] Campbell Clinic Department of Orthopaedic Surgery & Biomedical Engineering University of Tennessee, 956 Court Avenue, Memphis, TN 32116, USA
* Corresponding author.
E-mail address: kjsaleh@gmail.com

that might interfere with the fast-track protocols. General anesthesia, if used, will be done with sevoflurane and fentanyl in addition to peripheral nerve blocks.[7] Short-acting anesthetics such as propofol are always preferred.[6] Most patients undergoing THA and included in an enhanced recovery protocol (ERP) were operated under regional anesthesia, and general anesthesia was only indicated when peripheral nerve block failed to assure complete muscle relaxation or optimal analgesia.[6]

Spinal Anesthesia

Regional anesthesia allows for less narcotic administration, which has been associated with decreased postoperative nausea and hypotension. Regional anesthesia was mostly preferred. Low-dose spinal anesthesia (12.5 mg of isobaric bupivacaine) will not interfere with patients stay in the postanesthesia care unit (PACU) after THA.

Perioperative Pain Management

Pain affects patient stay after elective THA.[1] An early initiation of preemptive oral analgesia protocol is essential to shorten length of stay (LOS). Multimodal methods have been described including systemic analgesia, local joint infiltration with local anesthetic, and peripheral nerve blocks.

Several types of systemic analgesia are offered to patients in the perioperative setting including acetaminophen, nonsteroidal anti-inflammatory drugs (NSAIDs), opioids, and gabapentanoids. Acetaminophen is used widely in outpatient THA, either orally or intravenously.[7] Multiple protocols have been described, 975 mg orally every 6 hours, or 2 g for preoperative premedication and then every 12 hours.[7,8]

NSAIDs are also used as preemptive oral analgesics in addition to acetaminophen. Celebrex (cyclooxygenase-2-inhibitor) is commonly used with 400 mg given 1 hour prior to surgery and then postoperatively every 6 hours.[6] For fast-track THA, opioids are used as a rescue analgesic method. Their prescription as requested depends either on visual analog scale (VAS) scores or on numeric rating scale (NRS) scores that range from 0 to 10, with 10 being the worst possible pain. Avoiding systemic opioids decreases incidence of potential LOS-prolonging side effects such as respiratory depression, sedation, urine retention, nausea, vomiting, and pruritus. Ondansetron is often administered preoperatively to anticipate possible postoperative nausea and vomiting. A second antiemetic dose is given in the PACU to reinforce its effect.[6]

As part of a multimodal regimen, studies suggest oxycodone 5 mg will be administered orally (VAS<4). After a reevaluation and if VAS is greater than 7, oxycodone 10 mg or morphine 2 to 4 mg intravenously will be given. If VAS ranges between 4 and 7, however, another 5 mg of oxycodone will be prescribed.

Gabapentinoids are also used for their opioid-sparing effects, and to avoid narcotics side effects such as nausea, vomiting, and urinary retention. Recently, gabapentin has been an integral part of the multimodal analgesia concept for its antiallodynic and antihyperalgesic effect. Tiippana and colleagues[9] reported a 20% to 62% decrease in opioid consumption during the first 24 hours postoperatively when using a single dose of gabapentin. They also reported better pain control with gabapentinoids compared with placebo. Although there are no clear protocols on gabapentinoid administration, most studies used gabapentin or pregabalin 1 to 2 hours prior to surgery, and the doses ranged between 300 and 1200 mg with no additional side effects except minor sedation. A summary table of aforementioned medications is provided in Table 1.

Locally Infiltrative Analgesics

Local analgesic infiltration in patients undergoing THA has been reported to decrease not only pain scores postoperatively but also opioid consumption compared with placebo.[10] Different medications with different regimens have been used in local infiltration. Emerson and colleagues,[11] in a comparative study between standard bupivicaine wound infiltration and liposomal bupivacaine infiltration, reported that VAS scores were significantly lower in the liposomal group. Opioid doses along with total opioid consumption were also lower in the liposomal group. Local infiltration is a safe and simple method used as part of multimodal pain management following THA to decrease LOS and avoid opioid side effects. The conventional cocktails used in locally infiltrative injections usually contain 2 or more antalgic agents, such as opioids (eg, morphine, fentanyl, and codeine), NSAIDs (eg, diclofenac sodium, ibuprofen, and meloxicam), steroid hormones (eg, dexamethasone and betamethasone), and local anesthetics of amide derivatives (eg, bupivacaine and ropivacaine).

Peripheral Nerve Blocks

Peripheral nerve blocks have been described as part of fast-track surgery to promote early mobilization, rehabilitation, and decreased LOS. Ilfeld

Table 1 Analgesia modalities for outpatient total hip arthroplasty	
Acetaminophen	Dosage: 975 mg orally every 6 h, or 2 g for preoperative premedication and then every 12 h
NSAIDs	Example and dosage: Celebrex (Cyclooxygenase-2-Inhibitor) with 400 mg given 1 hour prior to surgery and then postoperatively every 6 h
Opioids (strictly for rescue analgesia)	Their prescription as requested depends either on VAS scores or on NRS scores that range from 0 to 10, with 10 being the worst possible pain Example and dosage: As part of a multimodal regimen, studies suggest oxycodone 5 mg will be administered orally (VAS<4) After a reevaluation and if VAS > 7, oxycodone 10 mg or morphine 2–4 mg intravenously will be given VAS ranges between 4–7; another 5 mg of oxycodone will be prescribed
Gabapentinoids	Example and dosage: Gabapentin or Pregabalin 1–2 h prior to surgery; dosage ranges between 300 and 1200 mg

and colleagues[7] considered the possibility of an overnight stay following THA, using ambulatory continuous psoas compartment nerve block with an at-home infusion pump. Multiple types of blocks have been described in the literature. Although the effectiveness of femoral nerve block and sciatic nerve block made approaches attractive, they do pose challenges in prolonging wait time and delay into getting to the operating room and starting physical therapy. Additionally, there have been some studies suggesting that regional anesthesia may be associated with fall risks. Conversely, Memtsoudis and colleagues[12] compared the rates of inpatient falls after a TKA. The study found that 10.9% of the patients had received neuraxial anesthetic; 12.9% of patients had received combined neuraxial/general anesthesia, and 76.2% of patients had general anesthesia.

Furthermore, nerve blocks provide an option for reducing dependence on parenteral opioids and helping prevent initiation of the pain cascade. Continuous femoral block and epidural block proved their efficacy, decreasing postoperative pain scores with no additional drowsiness compared with opioids.[13]

A study comparing outcomes in 100 patients undergoing total hip or knee arthroplasty who received a new total joint regional anesthesia (TJRA) protocol with 100 matched patients who received intravenous PCA with subsequent conversion to oral analgesics demonstrated improved pain control with the TJRA protocol on postoperative day 0 through postoperative day 3.3. The proportion of patients able to ambulate and meet the criteria for hospital discharge on postoperative days 1 through 3 was also significantly higher than the proportion of control patients who were able to ambulate.

Pulsed Electromagnetic Fields

Pulsed electromagnetic field (PEMF) stimulation is a safe and noninvasive therapy that enhances endogenous bone repair and reduces inflammatory process.[14] PEMF acts as adeonosine agonists of A2a receptors of inflammatory cells. As such, PEMF provides a strong anti-inflammatory effect and reduces the need for pain control medications, joint swelling, and the time to recovery.[15] A randomized control trial by Dallari and colleagues[15] investigated 30 patients undergoing hip revision. The subjects were treated for 6 hours per day up to 90 days after revision. Results of Dual Energy X-ray Absorptiometry (DXA) scans at Gruen zones suggested that the patients undergoing active stimulation developed higher bone mineral density responses at the medial cortex compared with control patients.[15] The authors further suggested that the PEMF helped improve functional recovery and bone stock.[15] Although PEMF has demonstrated postoperative success in aforementioned studies, it was first reported by Heylings and McMillin in 1988 as a preoperative treatment for patients awaiting primary THA. Heylings and McMillin correlated patients who had 3 or more sessions of PEMF with improved outcomes, fewer analgesics, and less disturbed sleep. They advocated utilization of PEMF as a method to improve movement and fitness prior to surgery. Such methodology may help improve ERPs regarding primary THA.[16]

INTRAOPERATIVE CONSIDERATIONS FOR OUTPATIENT TOTAL HIP ARTHROPLASTY

Operating Room Staff Management

Operating room efficiency is critical for successful implementation of an outpatient THA protocol. An operating room staff that is dedicated to joint reconstruction can increase room throughput while maintaining high-value care.[17,18] Additionally, specialized reconstruction teams assigned to a specific surgeon have been shown to improve efficiency.[19] Evidence suggests that the number of personnel in the operating room is directly related to procedure time, with approximately 34 minutes added to a procedure for each additional person present during the operation. Staff turnover is also identified as a potential source for increasing operating time, as well as safety compromise. Generally, traffic flow increases with a greater presence of individuals in the operating room, and this also may be a risk for postoperative infection due to air contamination. Therefore, the authors recommend intraoperative room efficiency may be optimized by minimizing staff turnover, traffic flow, and the size of the surgical team.

Surgical Intervention

Minimally invasive THA in combination with multimodal anesthesia techniques within rapid rehabilitation protocols often yields favorable results. The surgical approach is an imperative component of the outpatient THA procedure. Although the decision to pursue a specific approach depends on the patient-doctor relationship, and ultimately surgeon assessment, several surgeons have reported various procedures for successful outpatient arthroplasty. There remain more common approaches reported in literature regarding outpatient THA such as the modified Watson-Jones approach, the mini-posterior approach, and the 2-incision approach.

For most procedures a Foley catheter is inserted in the operating room, and intravenous antibiotics are started. Patients generally receive a titrated dose of for sedation during the procedure. Nausea prophylaxis is achieved with intravenous ondansetron hydrochloride and metoclopramide. Patients are to be given adequate hydration and assured to be preoperatively optimized.

Modified Watson-Jones Approach

The modified Watson-Jones approach is among the more commonly used approaches for quicker recovery in same-day THA pathways.[20,21] The modified approach uses an abductor-sparing anterolateral approach through the Watson-Jones interval.[20,21] The patient is positioned in lateral decubitus position using a standard table-mounted pelvic positioner. The posterior lower half of the table is removed, allowing for the operative leg to be placed in extension, adduction, and externa rotation.[20,21] A leg holder is used to support the operative leg in a position of 15° of abduction during the approach.[20,21]

The anterior border of the femur and the superior border of the greater trochanter are identified and marked.[20,21] The surgeon identifies the interval between the tensor fascia lata (TFL) and the gluteus medius and begins the incision.[20,21] The proximal end of the curvilinear incision begins slightly posterior to the interval, and curves toward the anterior superior aspect of the greater trochanter.[20,21] The incision then follows distally slightly posterior to the anterior border of the femur. Chen and Berger[22] describe that the incision is aimed to be no more than 3.5 to 4 inches long. Electrocautery maintains hemostasis as the surgeon dissects through fat down to the level of the fascia in line with the incision.[20,21] The border between the TFL and gluteus medius is identified. The incision is made over the anterior border of the gluteus medius and anterior to the greater trochanter.[20,21] A curved Hohmann retractor is placed over the capsule and superior aspect of the femoral neck under the gluteus medius and minimus.[20,21] The abductor muscle group is protected, and a lit retractor is placed inferior to the femoral neck. The retractors are spread; the anterior capsule is identified, and capsulotomy is performed. Chen and Berger suggest meticulous clearance of capsular debris along the saddle point between the greater trochanter and base of the femoral neck, because this identifies the superolateral border of the femoral neck osteotomy.[20,21]

The femoral head and neck are cut without hip dislocation. Using an oscilatting saw, the femoral head is cut into wafer slices.[20,21] The fragments are removed with a Kocher clamp and osteotome, allowing the tension in the hip joint to decrease. Chen and Berger suggest that the surgeon be mindful not to plunge to into the acetabulum with the oscillating saw. After the head is removed, the neck is cut to the templated level. Chen and Berger suggest placement of a lit, double pronged Mueller-type retractor beneath the lesser trochanter.[20,21] The surgeon then places the leg in a figure-of-4 position, with the foot placed into the hip pouch as the hip is flexed and externally rotated. The curved Hohmann retractor is designed to protect the abductors during the neck osteotomy, as an oscillating saw is used to perform the neck cut from to the templated level above the lesser trochanter.[20,21]

The acetabulum is prepared after the leg is taken out of the hip pouch and placed into the leg holder.[20,21] The double-pronged retractor is placed behind the acetabular wall, allowing the femur to be posteriorly retracted.[20,21] A cobra retractor is placed inferior to the obturator foramen, and a lit wide curved Hohmann retractor is placed posterosuperiorly to retract the abductor complex.[20,21] The acetabulum is visualized, and the labrum and pulvinar are excised.[20,21] The acetabulum is then reamed with cutout reamers. Chen and Berger report that the reaming should be conducted medially to the floor of the cotyloid fossa until a good press fit is achieved. The final implant is then impacted in appropriate positioning with or without screw fixation, followed by placement of a liner.[20,21]

The leg is then placed into a sterile kangaroo pouch attached to an assistant's gown.[20,21] This allows the hip to be manipulated for femoral preparation. The hip is extended, adducted, and externally rotated.[20,21] A curved Hohmann retractor is placed into the piriformis fossa over the greater trochanter. The placement of this retractor allows the surgeon to elevate the femur and retract the abductors posteriorly.[20,21] A double prolonged retractor is placed along the lateral aspect of the femur.[20,21] The posterior superior capsule is released from the saddle point, and the inner aspect of the greater trochanter.[20,21] After exposure is achieved, a curved awl enters the femoral canal. A large motorized burr is used to ream the inner aspect of the greater trochanter. A tapered femoral stem or a cylindrical stem may be used with this approach. Broaching is performed with offset handles until adequate fit is achieved.[20,21] The final stem is inserted, upon which a trial reduction is performed. The surgeon then assesses hip stability, soft tissue tension, and leg length. The trial head is then removed; the final head is placed, and the joint is then reduced.[20,21]

POSTOPERATIVE CARE
Postoperative Urinary Retention
Postoperative urine retention (POUR) is a common complication seen in THA. The incidence of POUR ranges from 0% to 75% of THA.[23,24] Pharmacologic methods have been attempted to avoid POUR, but results are inconclusive.[24]

Currently, intermittent bladder catheterization is the only option for prevention and treatment of POUR.[25] Utilization of indwelling catheterization is not recommended, as there is greater risk for urinary tract infection, as well as prosthesis infection and renal impairment.[26] POUR may prevent early mobilization and prolong hospital stay; therefore orthopedic surgeons should facilitate restoration of bladder function by using pain management protocols with opioid-sparing analgesia.[26]

Rehabilitation
Numerous improvements in both surgical and anesthesia techniques, including minimized soft-tissue dissection, implant improvements, multimodal analgesia, and blood management protocols have allowed patients undergoing THA to walk earlier with minimal pain. With such advances in orthopedic surgery, some surgeons have suggested that informal home exercise may be sufficient for most patients and offers substantial cost savings. It is estimated that approximately 40% of costs for a THA occur in the postdischarge setting, largely due to rehabilitation services.[22,27]

Discharge disposition also accounts for variability in recovery and rehabilitation after primary THA. In a retrospective study by Fu and colleagues,[28] researchers reviewed American College of Surgeons National Surgical Quality Improvement Program (NSQIP) data from 2011 to 2014. Researchers analyzed data from 54,837 THA cases to identify that patients discharged to continued inpatient care after THA were more likely to have septic complications, urinary complications, readmission, wound complications, and respiratory complications.[28] As such, a recent effort has been placed on dismissing formal physical therapy after total hip arthroplasty.

In a single-center randomized trial, Austin and colleagues assessed 120 patients undergoing primary THA who were eligible for home discharge. The experimental group was given a self-directed exercise regimen for 10 weeks, whereas the control group received a standard in-home and outpatient physical therapy protocol (2 weeks in-home physical therapy and 8 weeks of outpatient physical therapy). Researchers reported no significant difference between functional outcomes of patients receiving formal therapy and those receiving unsupervised home exercise.

Although a recent effort has been placed toward in-home physical therapy protocols, conventional therapy warrants discussion.

Regardless of how it is done, perioperative therapy propagates healing following arthroplasty. Studies have shown that patients who do not receive rehabilitation following THA will develop functional limitations within 1 year after surgery.[29,30] Physiotherapy improves strength, gait, and speed after THA and helps prevent complications such as thromboembolic disease. In addition, physiotherapy increases the patient's mobility and offers education regarding exercises and precautions necessary for hospitalization and discharge. Improved rehabilitation following outpatient THA has been proposed as major factors to shorter LOS and earlier ambulation.[31] No consensus exists for the most effective physiotherapy in primary THA.

A randomized clinical trial by Umpierres and colleagues[32] assessed 2 different types of physiotherapy protocols. One cohort of patients received verbal instructions and physiotherapy exercise demonstrations. The other cohort received the same instructions and demonstration associated with daily practice guided by a physiotherapist.[32] The outcomes were assessed 15 days postoperatively in 106 patients.[32] Researchers reported that the physiotherapist-guided cohort displayed higher muscle strength, force scores, and degrees in range of motion than the nonassisted cohort. Researchers concluded that there is likely a benefit with physiotherapist involvement in primary THA with regard to functional capacity and mobility.[32]

Kerr and Kohan reported a postoperative protocol aimed at mobilizing all patients within 3 to 4 hours after surgery. Patients were required to walk again every 2 to 3 hours after surgery. A fluid bolus (200–300 mL) was given prior to the patient standing for the first time. Patients were encouraged to walk at least 30 minutes. Patients were encouraged to walk independently with crutches, followed by self-mobilization without the crutches.[33]

SUMMARY

The authors provided a literature update regarding development of outpatient THA protocols. Outpatient THA has potential for more rapid recovery and return to function for eligible candidates. Careful patient selection, implementation of newer anesthetic and rehabilitation protocols, and minimally invasive approaches to THA all play a role in outpatient care pathways. The general concept remains that each process, whether pre-, intra-, or postoperative, holds tremendous value for patients involved in the care continuum. Although no gold standard pathway exists, it is clear that further evidence is needed to provide surgeons with examples on how to conduct such procedures at their respective institutions.

REFERENCES

1. Husted H, Lunn TH, Troelsen A, et al. Why still in hospital after fast-track hip and knee arthroplasty? Acta Orthop 2011;82(6):679–84.
2. Molko S, Combalia A. Rapid recovery programmes for hip and knee arthroplasty. An update. Rev Esp Cir Ortop Traumatol 2017;61(2):130–8.
3. Berger RA, Kusuma SK, Sanders SA, et al. The feasibility and perioperative complications of outpatient knee arthroplasty. Clin Orthop Relat Res 2009; 467(6):1443–9.
4. Berger RA, Sanders S, D'Ambrogio E, et al. Minimally invasive quadriceps-sparing TKA: results of a comprehensive pathway for outpatient TKA. J Knee Surg 2006;19(2):145–8.
5. Berger RA, Sanders S, Gerlinger T, et al. Outpatient total knee arthroplasty with a minimally invasive technique. J Arthroplasty 2005;20(7 Suppl 3): 33–8.
6. Berger RA, Sanders SA, Thill ES, et al. Newer anesthesia and rehabilitation protocols enable outpatient hip replacement in selected patients. Clin Orthop Relat Res 2009;467(6):1424–30.
7. Ilfeld BM, Gearen PF, Enneking FK, et al. Total hip arthroplasty as an overnight-stay procedure using an ambulatory continuous psoas compartment nerve block: a prospective feasibility study. Reg Anesth Pain Med 2006;31(2):113–8.
8. Lunn TH, Kristensen BB, Gaarn-Larsen L, et al. Post-anaesthesia care unit stay after total hip and knee arthroplasty under spinal anaesthesia. Acta Anaesthesiol Scand 2012;56(9):1139–45.
9. Tiippana EM, Hamunen K, Kontinen VK, et al. Do surgical patients benefit from perioperative gabapentin/pregabalin? A systematic review of efficacy and safety. Anesth Analg 2007;104(6):1545–56. Table of contents.
10. Jimenez-Almonte JH, Wyles CC, Wyles SP, et al. Is local infiltration analgesia superior to peripheral nerve blockade for pain management after THA: a network meta-analysis. Clin Orthop Relat Res 2016;474(2):495–516.
11. Emerson RH, Barrington JW, Olugbode O, et al. Comparison of local infiltration analgesia to bupivacaine wound infiltration as part of a multimodal pain program in total hip replacement. J Surg orthopaedic Adv 2015;24(4):235–41.
12. Memtsoudis SG, Danninger T, Rasul R, et al. Inpatient falls after total knee arthroplasty: the role of anesthesia type and peripheral nerve blocks. Anesthesiology 2014;120(3):551–63.

13. Nishio S, Fukunishi S, Juichi M, et al. Comparison of continuous femoral nerve block, caudal epidural block, and intravenous patient-controlled analgesia in pain control after total hip arthroplasty: a prospective randomized study. Orthop Rev 2014;6(1):5138.

14. Zorzi C, Dall'Oca C, Cadossi R, et al. Effects of pulsed electromagnetic fields on patients' recovery after arthroscopic surgery: prospective, randomized and double-blind study. Knee Surg Sports Traumatol Arthrosc 2007;15(7):830–4.

15. Dallari D, Fini M, Giavaresi G, et al. Effects of pulsed electromagnetic stimulation on patients undergoing hip revision prostheses: a randomized prospective double-blind study. Bioelectromagnetics 2009;30(6):423–30.

16. Heylings DJA MW. Pulsed electromagnetic fields as an analgesic in osteoarthritis of the hip joint. Paper presented at: Procs British Association of Clinical Anatomists Conference. London (UK), December 1988.

17. Small TJ, Gad BV, Klika AK, et al. Dedicated orthopedic operating room unit improves operating room efficiency. J Arthroplasty 2013;28(7):1066–71. e1062.

18. Marjamaa RA, Torkki PM, Hirvensalo EJ, et al. What is the best workflow for an operating room? A simulation study of five scenarios. Health Care Manag Sci 2009;12(2):142–6.

19. Attarian DE, Wahl JE, Wellman SS, et al. Developing a high-efficiency operating room for total joint arthroplasty in an academic setting. Clin Orthop Relat Res 2013;471(6):1832–6.

20. Hu CC, Chern JS, Hsieh PH, et al. Two-incision versus modified Watson-Jones total hip arthroplasty in the same patients– a prospective study of clinical outcomes and patient preferences. Chang Gung Med J 2012;35(1):54–61.

21. Chen D, Berger RA. Outpatient minimally invasive total hip arthroplasty via a modified Watson-Jones approach: technique and results. Instr Course Lect 2013;62:229–36.

22. Lavernia CJ, Villa JM. Rapid recovery programs in arthroplasty: the money side. J Arthroplasty 2015;30(4):533–4.

23. Balderi T, Carli F. Urinary retention after total hip and knee arthroplasty. Minerva Anestesiol 2010;76(2):120–30.

24. Baldini G, Bagry H, Aprikian A, et al. Postoperative urinary retention: anesthetic and perioperative considerations. Anesthesiology 2009;110(5):1139–57.

25. Madersbacher H, Cardozo L, Chapple C, et al. What are the causes and consequences of bladder overdistension? ICI-RS 2011. Neurourol Urodyn 2012;31(3):317–21.

26. Kehlet H. Fast-track hip and knee arthroplasty. Lancet 2013;381(9878):1600–2.

27. Ong KL, Lotke PA, Lau E, et al. Prevalence and costs of rehabilitation and physical therapy after primary TJA. J Arthroplasty 2015;30(7):1121–6.

28. Fu MC, Samuel AM, Sculco PK, et al. Discharge to inpatient facilities after total hip arthroplasty is associated with increased postdischarge morbidity. J Arthroplasty 2017;32(9S):S144–9.

29. Trudelle-Jackson E, Smith SS. Effects of a late-phase exercise program after total hip arthroplasty: a randomized controlled trial. Arch Phys Med Rehabil 2004;85(7):1056–62.

30. Okoro T, Lemmey AB, Maddison P, et al. An appraisal of rehabilitation regimes used for improving functional outcome after total hip replacement surgery. Sports Med Arthrosc Rehabil Ther Technol 2012;4(1):5.

31. Lovald S, Ong K, Lau E, et al. Patient selection in outpatient and short-stay total knee arthroplasty. J Surg orthopaedic Adv 2014;23(1):2–8.

32. Umpierres CS, Ribeiro TA, Marchisio AE, et al. Rehabilitation following total hip arthroplasty evaluation over short follow-up time: randomized clinical trial. J Rehabil Res Dev 2014;51(10):1567–78.

33. Kerr DR, Kohan L. Local infiltration analgesia: a technique for the control of acute postoperative pain following knee and hip surgery: a case study of 325 patients. Acta Orthop 2008;79(2):174–83.

Impact of Outpatient Total Joint Replacement on Postoperative Outcomes

Danielle Lovett-Carter, MD[a], Zain Sayeed, MD, MHA[a],
Leila Abaab, MD[a,b], Vinay Pallekonda, MD[b],
William Mihalko, MD, PhD[c],
Khaled J. Saleh, MD, MSc, FRCS(C), MHCM, CPE[a],*

KEYWORDS

- Outpatient total joint arthroplasty • Total knee arthroplasty • Total hip arthroplasty
- Length of stay • Readmission • Outcomes • Cost • Patient-reported outcome measures

KEY POINTS

- The success of fast-track pathways in Europe and the United States is a strong indicator that outpatient joint replacement will soon be offered more widely and will be recognized by patients and surgeons as a safe option.
- Younger patients with a lower body mass index and fewer comorbidities are appropriate candidates for outpatient hip and knee arthroplasty.
- Outpatient arthroplasty in the proper patients has comparable, if not superior, outcomes compared with standard inpatient arthroplasty.

INTRODUCTION

Annual demand for total joint arthroplasty (TJA) has been steadily increasing over the past 30 years and is projected to continue to increase substantially over the coming years as life expectancy and obesity increase and surgical technique and perioperative management are optimized.[1] With continuous growth, surgeons and hospitals have sought to improve quality of joint replacement while simultaneously aiming at lowering cost and resource utilization. This effort has centered on the development of clinical care pathways and perioperative standardized protocols aimed at optimizing postoperative outcomes, including hospital length of stay, complications, and readmissions, among others. Over the past several

years, there has been a growing trend in the literature toward early patient discharge.

The leading cause of 30-day readmission after total knee arthroplasty (TKA) is deep or superficial surgical site infection (SSI), which accounts for 12.1% of unplanned readmissions.[2,3] SSIs accounted for 23.5% of unplanned readmissions in total hip arthroplasty (THA) patients, just behind hip dislocation, according to one report. Ong and colleagues[4] report length of hospital stay is implicated as a risk factor for SSI or prosthetic joint infection, among others such as comorbidities, sex and duration of procedure. Furthermore, SSIs have been shown to double length of hospital stay by a median of 2 weeks, which further drives up associated costs.[5]

Hospital stay for TKA has decreased from 9 days to 4 days on average[6] and for THA, from

Funding Sources: No additional funding sources were used for this article.
Conflicts of Interest: No conflicts of interest are evident for authors of this article.
[a] Department of Orthopaedics, Detroit Medical Center, 4201 St Antoine Street, Detroit, MI 48201, USA; [b] Department of Anesthesiology – NorthStar Anesthesia, Detroit Medical Center, 4201 St Antoine Street, Detroit, MI 48201, USA; [c] Campbell Clinic Department of Orthopaedic Surgery & Biomedical Engineering University of Tennessee, 956 Court Avenue, Memphis, TN 32116, USA
* Corresponding author.
E-mail address: kjsaleh@gmail.com

4.6 days to 2.9 days at 1 center.[7] These proto-cols have aimed at standardizing procedure, pain control, education, and early rehabilitation and implement preventative measures for com-plications. This trend toward decreasing length of hospital stay has led to the development of pathways that allow medically and socially opti-mized patients to undergo TJA in an outpatient setting. Although some studies have shown promise in using this method, the results may not be generally applied.

The aim of this review is to determine if outpa-tient TJA leads to similar outcomes as standard-stay inpatients. Postoperative outcomes may be assessed by pain, same-day discharge, complica-tions, readmissions, reoperation, patient satisfac-tion, patient-reported outcomes (PROs), and cost.

METHODS

The authors performed searches in electronic da-tabases (Embase, PubMed, Web of Science, and Cochrane) to identify eligible studies published before April 2017. Exact search term used were "total hip replacement" OR "total hip arthro-plasty" OR "THA" OR "THR", "total knee replacement" OR "total knee arthroplasty" OR "TKA" OR "TKR", "total joint replacement" OR "total joint arthroplasty" OR "TJR" OR "TJA", "outpatient", and "outcomes" OR "postopera-tive outcomes." Duplicates were removed.

To be considered for inclusion in this review, studies must have included a cohort of patients who underwent outpatient TKA or THA. Unfortu-nately, the definition of outpatient varied among investigators. The vast majority agreed outpa-tient meant patients were discharged to home on the same day as the surgery; however, 1 article considered discharge at 23 hours postoperatively or less acceptable. Studies were excluded if pa-tients stayed more than 24 hours or if they comprised only patients undergoing partial or single-component joint replacement. A total of 14 studies was identified from the literature as meeting criteria and were included in the review.

RESULTS AND DISCUSSION

Nine studies examined outcomes in outpatient THA and 6 in outpatient TKA (with 1 study covering both). Of the studies that compared groups prospectively, sample size tended to be low and thus more difficult to generalize. Because outpatient total joint replacement is a relatively new concept, researchers are reach-ing the end of a process of carrying out small-scale studies and case series to determine

procedure safety and moving toward larger-scale randomized trials to refine protocol de-tails. Based on the evidence compiled in this re-view, only 1 randomized controlled trial (RCT) was carried out. Larger-scale, multicenter ran-domized trials are needed to determine exactly which candidates will benefit from this inter-vention as well as how best to implement outpatient joint protocols. Outcomes for TJA included same-day discharge, postoperative pain, complications, readmissions, reopera-tions, PROs, and cost.

TOTAL HIP ARTHROPLASTY OUTCOMES

Nine studies ranged from level I evidence to level IV (Table 1). Goyal and colleagues[8] are the only investigators who carried out an RCT (level I). Aynardi and colleagues[9] compared 119 patients who underwent outpatient THA with 78 inpatients undergoing the same proced-ure by the same surgeon but these groups were not randomly assigned. Similarly, Springer and colleagues[10] retrospectively compared THA in-patients with outpatients nonrandomly. Bertin[11] examined patient outcomes from a financial aspect, which falls under economic and decision analysis (level IV). The remaining 5 studies were case series in nature (Dorr and colleagues,[12] Berger and colleagues,[13] Berger and col-leagues,[14] Berger,[15] and Den Hartog and col-leagues[16]) and looked at outcomes from a cohort of patients without comparing them to a similar group.

Same-Day Discharge

All investigators who carried out prospective studies used length of stay or same-day discharge as an outcome. For the THA patients, Goyal and colleagues[8] achieved a 76% rate of same-day discharge, and all but 1 of the remain-ing patients left the following day. Interestingly, 18 of the 108 patients randomized to the inpa-tient group met the same-day discharge criteria and chose to leave after their surgery. This was not the only report of difficulty with randomiza-tion, which may be an issue in smaller, single-center studies. Berger and colleagues[13] reported that their team had attempted to randomize the patients but ultimately had to abandon the idea after many patients requested overnight hospitalization and many more requested to be part of the study despite not being selected. For this reason, their rate of same-day discharge was 100%. The same inves-tigators had similar success with older studies, achieving a rate of 85% discharge in both 2004

Table 1
Total hip arthroplasty outcomes

Study	Level of Evidence	Sample	Rate of SDD (%)	Surgical Approach	Readmissions	Emergency Department Visits	Complications	Cost
Goyal et al,[8] 2017	Level I RCT	112	76	Direct ant approach	4/112	2 ED visits 2 reoperations	2 reoperations	—
Aynardi et al,[9] 2014	Level III Case-control	119	93	Direct ant approach	0/119	—	No complications	$6800 < inpatient
Springer et al,[10] 2017	Level III Case-control	77	100	Posterolateral approach	0/77	1 ED visit	No complications	—
Bertin,[11] 2005	Level IV Financial analysis	—	—	Posterolateral approach	—	—	—	$6500 < inpatient
Dorr et al,[12] 2010	Level IV Case series	69	77	Post mini-incision approach	0/69	—	No complications	—
Berger et al,[13] 2009	Level IV Case series	150	100	Minimally invasive THA	3/150	9 ED visits	2 fractures 1 pneumonia	—
Berger et al,[14] 2004	Level IV Case series	100	85	Minimally invasive THA	0/100	—	No complications	—
Berger et al,[15] 2003	Level IV Case series	88	85	Minimally invasive THA	0/88	—	No complications	—
Den Hartog et al,[16] 2015	Level IV Case series	27	89	Direct ant approach	1/27	—	1 seroma	—

Abbreviation: SDD, same day discharge.

and 2003 reports. Dorr and colleagues[12] had a similar rate of same-day discharge at 77%. All but 4 of Aynardi and colleagues'[9] cohort of 119 were discharged on the day of surgery (93%) and 24 of Den Hartog and colleagues'[16] group of 27 (89%).

When considering same-day discharge as an outcome, these results must be taken with some understanding. Lack of randomization leaves room for selection bias, which most investigators recognized. The vast majority of investigators hand-selected younger, healthier patients for outpatient procedures and many participants, in turn, also had to self-select their outpatient status. So not only were the surgeons identifying a low-risk population but also they were further stratifying only those that had the potential confidence, social support, access to services, and resilience to be discharged after a TJA, traditionally an inpatient procedure.

This issue raises some other important points for discussion, such as why patients who requested an overnight stay are fearful of outpatient surgery. The authors[12] identified through patient feedback that the largest barriers for same-day discharge were fear of uncontrolled pain and fear of dependency on others.[12] Many patient misconceptions can be easily overcome through education, and these factors are vital to the development of a successful comprehensive clinical pathway for outpatient joint replacement.

All prospective studies in this review included a form of standardized protocols for outpatient TKA or THA. This ranged from standardization of surgical technique, anesthesia, management of postoperative pain, nausea, and hypotension to rehabilitation protocol and patient education. These clinical protocols required commitment of the multidisciplinary team to the goal of same-day discharge. This meant prompt responses from nursing and physical therapists to postoperative issues to achieve this goal; thus, a committed team, as many articles rightfully pointed out, was a vital part of the process. Because outpatient TJA is still a relatively new exploit, however, it is unknown which protocols are superior and cost effective.

Berger and colleagues[13] were among the investigators who detailed one such clinical protocol, which includes a description of preoperative, intraoperative, and postoperative care and required the combined effort of a multidisciplinary team. In the case of Den Hartog and colleagues,[16] the investigators were building on an already established fast-track protocol that was in place at their hospital. This protocol was developed from 2009 to 2011, with every step of the process developed from evidence-based practice, from preoperative education to follow-up. This study, carried out at a large teaching hospital, showed that when this rapid recovery protocol was implemented, there was a decrease in hospital stay for unselected primary THA patients without any change in complication rate, readmission rate, or reoperation rate. Several other hospitals have been implementing similar protocols with success in Europe, such as Winther and colleagues'[17] in Norway. Both Berger[13] and Den Hartog's[16] protocols were similar in some ways and differed in others, proving that there may be variations in the protocol while still achieving desired outcomes. The success of these pathways in Europe and the United States is a strong indicator that outpatient joint replacement will soon be offered more widely and will be recognized by patients and surgeons as a safe option.

Postoperative Pain

Few studies considered postoperative pain as an outcome measure. Den Hartog and colleagues'[16] cohort saw a statistically significant reduction in pain using the numeric rating scale (NRS); however, no control group was available. Goyal and colleagues[8] used the visual analog scale as an outcome and found there was no difference in pain at baseline, on the day of surgery, or at 4 weeks. The outpatient THA group did report experiencing more pain on the first day after surgery, however. Whether this additional pain was causing problems, such as return to an office or emergency department (ED), is unclear.

Several factors may influence pain and one worth considering is surgical approach. Berger and colleagues[13–15] used a minimally invasive technique for THA that reduces damage to muscles and tendons.[18] Goyal and colleagues,[8] Den Hartog and colleagues,[16] and Aynardi and colleagues,[9] all used a direct anterior approach, which has been shown in the literature to be associated with less pain, a shorter hospital stay, and a shorter operative time.[19,20] It is more technically demanding, however, and has its own unique set of complications. Because this technique has a steeper learning curve, its role as an outpatient procedure may not be generalizable to all surgeons in all clinical settings. Bertin[11] and Springer and colleagues[10] reported using a posterolateral technique. Bertin[11] however, focused only on financial rather than patient outcomes. Springer and colleagues[10] reported no readmissions or complications for the 77 THA patients included in the study. And although this suggests this may be a successful approach for outpatients, because such a small number of the outpatient THA studies were carried out using the more traditional posterolateral approach, it is difficult to say definitively that it, too, would be feasible as an outpatient procedure.

Complications, Readmissions, and Reoperations

Another outcome of interest was the concept of safety and feasibility. Most investigators used readmissions, complications, and sometimes ED visits as measures for procedure safety. Of the 8 studies that looked at outpatient THA outcomes, there were a total of 820 patients and only 8 readmissions (<1%). Dorr and colleagues[12] and Berger and colleagues[14] reported no complications or readmissions at 6-month and 3-month follow-ups, respectively. Springer and colleagues[10] and Berger and colleagues[14] also noted no complications or readmissions postdischarge. Den Hartog and colleagues'[16] only complication was 1 readmission for seroma formation. Goyal and colleagues[8] and Aynardi and colleagues,[9] who both had an inpatient control group, demonstrated no difference in complications, readmission, or reoperation between inpatients and outpatients. The former saw 4 outpatients readmitted and 2 reoperations, whereas the latter reported none.

Berger and colleagues[13] saw 3 readmissions in 3 months. The first suffered a stress fracture at the distal femoral stem 6 weeks postoperatively; the others were for femoral fracture posttrauma and pneumonia (which subsequently was complicated by a psoas abscess). Overall, the rate of complications was exceptionally low. A study of more than 58,000 standard-stay primary hip arthroplasty patients showed that 3.9% suffered hip dislocation, 0.9% developed a pulmonary embolism, and 0.2% developed a deep SSI in the first 26 weeks.[21] The rate of adverse outcomes was highest in the hospitalization period and fell considerably on discharge. Because all complications of the studies discussed in this review occurred between 11 days and 3 months of surgery, it could be argued that the outpatient aspect of their experience played a minimal role in the complication and possibly prevented other complications. Their comparatively lower complication rate is also likely a result of the recruitment of younger, healthier patients.

Additionally, 3 studies recorded ED visits. Berger and colleagues[13] reported 9 ED visits without admission: 3 in the first week for dehydration, pain, and anemia requiring transfusion; 1 in the first month for benign leg swelling; and the remaining 5, which were unrelated to the surgery. Goyal and colleagues[8] reported 2 ED visits as well as 2 acute office visits before scheduled follow-up. Springer and colleagues[10] noted 1 ED visit from an outpatient THA patient. Reporting of ED visits is a new phenomenon, with most studies failing to mention it. It is a valuable outcome in terms of evaluating success of outpatient TJA, because it lends insight into potential issues with the outpatient protocol and how soon postoperatively these issues are arising. Although ED presentations in these studies were variable, the numbers are too few to make a determination. Furthermore, Berger and colleagues[13] are the only investigators who report reasons for representation. Future trials should include accounts of ED presentations and the reason for them to identify areas of weakness, for example, pain control or hydration.

When evaluating complications, it is also important to consider patients' baseline status. Berger and colleagues,[14] Berger,[15] Den Hartog and colleagues,[16] and Aynardi and colleagues[9] all used moderately strict criteria centering mostly around low-grade American Society of Anesthesiologists status, age, a desire to have same-day discharge, operative risk stratification, and home support. Berger and colleagues[13] as well as Springer and colleagues[10] had similar strict criteria to their outpatient TKA counterparts, excluding those with previous cardiopulmonary events, significant comorbidities, and body mass index (BMI) greater than 40. Dorr and colleagues[12] required only self-enrollment for outpatient surgery and age less than 65. Outcomes seemed uniform despite the variation in patient selection; however, it does not seem that any investigator offered outpatient THA to patients over 75 or those with significant comorbidities.

Patient-Reported Outcomes

PROs are a vital component of assessing the outcomes of TKA and THA.[22] Many PRO questionnaires are available that have been validated in this population, such as the Western Ontario and McMaster Universities Osteoarthritis Index, the Harris Hip Score (HHS), and the Forgotten Joint Score-12. Dorr and colleagues,[9] Berger and colleagues,[13] and Springer and colleagues[10] used patient satisfaction as an outcome. The former 2 found that 96% were satisfied with the decision to undergo outpatient surgery and would do so again, whereas the latter found no difference in satisfaction rates in outpatients compared with inpatients. A further 87% in Dorr and colleagues' study found that it gave them confidence. They were also asked to keep diaries and record their functional progress. Of the diaries that were returned, 82% had returned to independent activities of daily living, 84% were driving, and 98% were walking 1 mile at 3 weeks. Berger and colleagues[14] used the 36-Item Short Form Health Survey and the HHS and found a significant improvement in postoperative scores. The same investigators also looked at functional milestones, such as driving, returning to work, and so forth, similar to Dorr and colleagues.[9] Additionally, Dorr and colleagues,[9] Berger and colleagues,[13] and Goyal and colleagues[8] also used the HHS with improvement. Den Hartog and colleagues[16] included the EuroQol Quality of Life Scale (EQ-5D) assessment scale and the NRS for pain at rest and during activity. Springer and colleagues,[10] Bertin,[11] Berger,[15] and Aynardi and colleagues[9] did not use any PROs.

The use of PROs is arguably limited in the majority of these studies without a control group to a certain extent. Although they show statistically significant improvements, previous literature has already demonstrated that THA improves functional status for the majority of patients it is indicated for, regardless of how long they spend in hospital. These outcomes measures would be of far greater benefit if compared with a control group with a standard length stay to detect subtle functional differences. This is seen in the RCT by Goyal and colleagues,[8] where no difference was noted between the HHS of inpatients and outpatients at 4 weeks.

Dorr and colleagues'[9] and Berger and colleagues'[13] choice to include patient satisfaction and confidence, despite being a crude measure, is a little more specific to the outpatient component of the surgery and may have some value in terms of highlighting the need to combat fears and misconceptions about the procedure. This is explored in a qualitative study by Specht and colleagues,[23] who report that education on dealing with pain in short-stay TKA and THA patients is vital. Patients reported preoperative education on what to expect as well as having a well-planned schedule during hospitalization were important to them and contributed to overall satisfaction.

Cost

As the estimated number of THAs and TKAs is set to increase over the coming years, there will be an anticipated economic burden on health care facilities.[8] One potential way to decrease expenditure is to minimize hospital stay and ultimately make outpatient TJA a widespread option for suitable patients. Because outpatient TJA is being developed as part of a comprehensive protocol, several investigators looked at whether this was cost effective. Bertin[11] found that the average hospital bill was approximately $4000 less for outpatients and associated charges, such as home physical therapy, were $2500 less. Aynardi and colleagues[9] reported a similar saving where outpatient THA was approximately $6800 cheaper overall than the inpatient procedure. Another element to the cost section was an issue raised by Goyal and colleagues[8] regarding additional work for the staff involved with the surgeons' office. There have been anecdotal reports that outpatient THA caused many additional office calls and visits. The same investigators found this not to be the case, and they attribute the preoperative education program to lack of difference in staff work between inpatient and outpatient THA.

TOTAL KNEE ARTHROPLASTY OUTCOMES

All TKA studies included were between level II and level IV evidence, because no groups were randomized (Table 2). A study by Kolisek and colleagues[6] compared patients undergoing TKA as inpatients with those undergoing the same procedure as outpatients, prospectively. Similarly, Huang and colleagues[24] prospectively compared similar groups; however, the investigators' focus was on cost as opposed to surgical outcomes. Springer and colleagues[10] included both THA and TKA outpatients as part of a retrospective case-control study. Lovald and colleagues[25] reported a large-scale retrospective cohort, where the investigators compared characteristics and outcomes of patients undergoing TKA in terms of length of hospital stay. This ranged from outpatient procedures to 5 or more hospital days. Berger and colleagues[26] compared patients who underwent TKA as outpatients to patients who underwent outpatient UKA. And lastly, Berger and colleagues[27] performed a case series (level IV), where the investigators evaluated patient outcomes but did not compare them to another group.

Same-Day Discharge

Berger and colleagues[27] had a 98% success rate for same-day discharge and Berger and colleagues[26] had a rate of 94%. Kolisek and colleagues[6] had a discharge rate of 100%; however, these participants were discharged within 23 hours, not on the same day. Again, similar to the THA studies, no study randomized its participants, leaving room for selection bias

Table 2
Total knee arthroplasty outcomes

Study	Level of Evidence	Sample	Rate of SDD (%)	Surgical Approach	Readmissions	Emergency Department Visits	Complications	Cost
Kolisek et al,[6] 2009	Level II Prospective	150	100	Med parapatellar approach	4/150	—	2 reoperations	—
Huang et al,[24] 2016	Level III Case-control	20	100	—	0/20	—	No complications	30% < inpatient
Springer et al,[10] 2017	Level III Case-control	166	100	Med parapatellar approach	12/166	3 ED visit	No complications	—
Lovald et al,[25] 2014	Level III Retrospective cohort	454	100	—	4/454	—	9 DVTs 9 infections 2 dislocations 2 revisions 26 stiffness 144 joint pain	$8527 < inpatient
Berger et al,[26] 2009	Level III Case-control	86	94	Minimally invasive TKA	8/86	2 ED visits	2 SSIs 1 arthrofibrosis 1 DVT 2 anemias 1 GI bleed	—
Berger et al,[27] 2006	Level IV Case series	100	98	Minimally invasive TKA	2/100	—	1 SSI 1 Arthrofibrosis 1 GI bleed	—

and the other issues previously discussed with the THA group. Lovald and colleagues'[25] retrospective cohort showed that among a sample of 102,684 patients undergoing TKA, the percentage who made up outpatient procedures was less than 0.5%. The study reports that they only considered outpatients who were discharged routinely.

The majority of studies tended to favor strict or semistrict criteria for patient selection, such as Springer and colleagues,[10] Huang and colleagues,[24] and Kolisek and colleagues.[6] Berger and colleagues[27] did not enroll patients for same-day discharge if they had a high BMI, significant medical comorbidities, or a cardiopulmonary event in the past year. Only Berger and colleagues[26] allowed patients to select their own status as outpatient after TKA, regardless of age or BMI. Based on the high rate of same-day discharge, the outpatient TKA seems to be feasible in a range of patients, selected and unselected alike. As a stand-alone measure, however, this may not be useful because it needs to be taken in conjunction with readmission rates and ED visits.

Postoperative Pain

Lovald and colleagues[25] reported that in the first 90 days after TKA, those who underwent the procedure as outpatients had less pain and stiffness, with only 31% reporting pain in the joint compared with 43% in the short-stay and standard-stay groups. This review and the cost savings report by Huang and colleagues,[24] unfortunately, do not specify which surgical approach was used during the TKA or comment on the pain regimen implemented, which was likely different at every center.

For the outpatient TKA, Berger and colleagues[26,27] used a minimally invasive quadriceps-sparing technique. This has also been shown to reduce pain and hospital stay in the short term based on the principles of minimizing interruption and dissection of neurovascular tissues.[28] Kolisek and colleagues[6] and Springer and colleagues[10] both used a standard medial parapatellar approach. Both studies mentioned above did not use pain as an outcome measure so it is not possible to comment on whether the minimally invasive procedure does, in fact, reduce pain. All studies had similarly low numbers of readmissions and complications. Thus, it seems from the evidence discussed in this article that there were no major barriers to performing the standard TKA compared with the minimally invasive approach. Small sample size and a lack of outcome

measures used, however, make comparison difficult. Although readmission rates may be similar, other factors like pain, function, and satisfaction may vary in the short term.

Complications, Readmissions, and Reoperations

Of the 6 studies who reported on outpatient TKA outcomes, there were a total of 816 patients and 22 readmissions (2.7%). Lovald and colleagues[25] compared complications, readmissions, mortality, and rate of revision across outpatient, short-stay, standard-stay, and extended-stay patients using multivariate Cox regression analysis. Although pain and stiffness were improved in the outpatient and short-stay groups, the same groups had a higher rate of readmission and revision. The readmission rate for outpatient TKA was 0.9% compared with 0.6% for short-stay patients and 0.5% in standard-stay patients. The study reports that this cohort was more likely to be younger and have fewer comorbidities but does not comment on selection process for outpatient procedure. Because the patients are younger and healthier, it could be speculated that they are more active and more likely to engage in activity that causes mechanical problems with the prosthesis, which the investigators identified as one of the main reasons for revision. Lovald and colleagues[25] also speculated that given the recent studies showing success with outpatient TJA as a cost-saving measure, several institutes may be performing outpatient TKA without developing a standardized care pathway, leading to poor patient selection and higher readmission rates. Because the Lovald and colleagues review is on a much larger scale and follows outcomes at multiple centers for a longer time period, it highlights some interesting data that need to be further explored in a prospective manner.

Berger and colleagues[27] had 100 participants and saw 2 readmissions within the first few weeks for a cardiac event and a bleeding gastric ulcer as well as a further SSI and manipulation under anesthesia for arthrofibrosis. Berger and colleagues[26] reported 4 readmissions from the TKA group within the first week (2 for anemia, 1 for gastrointestinal [GI] bleed and 1 deep vein thrombosis [DVT]), 4 more within the first 3 months (2 SSIs, 1 GI bleed, and 1 admission for manipulation under anesthesia), and 2 visits to the ED for nausea and benign swelling. Based on these reports, the investigators note that readmissions may be higher in an unselected patient group and recommended a more stringent screening process.

Springer and colleagues,[10] however, who reported strict criteria excluding patients with active cardiopulmonary disease, history of sleep apnea, DVT, or pulmonary embolism, had similar numbers, with a 12% readmission rate for outpatient TKAs compared with 6% for inpatient TKAs as well as 3 ED visits, which was more than the inpatient TKA and all THA patients combined. The most common reasons for this included wound issues, inadequate pain control, or adverse reaction to pain medication. This report demonstrates that even in a select group, outpatient TKA does continue to show a trend toward a higher rate of readmissions and ED visits.

Patient-Reported Outcomes

Springer and colleagues[10] reported no difference in satisfaction between patients undergoing inpatient TKA compared with outpatient TKA. For the remainder of the studies, no investigators used PRO assessments. Kesterke and colleagues[22] reported that PRO assessments can be conducted electronically for all ages without difficulty and can be carried out quickly, such as in the waiting room before follow-up appointment. This reduces the issues with compliance when postal questionnaires are used. Future studies should incorporate appropriate PRO assessments because it is particularly important to collect longitudinal data when evaluating a procedure.[22]

Cost

Similar to the outpatient THA, the outpatient TKA has been shown to be a cost-saving procedure. A Canadian study by Huang and colleagues[24] demonstrated a savings of 30% of inpatient costs. Although a majority of savings came from the surgical floor care, there were also reductions in pharmacy costs and physiotherapy. Lovald and colleagues,[25] in a large-scale review of the US Medicare population, showed a mean savings of $8527 for the outpatient cases compared with the standard stay patients. And with Medicare paying for an estimated 55% of TKAs, this represents significant federal savings. The trend in these studies is that the outpatients tend to have fewer comorbidities and be younger, thus likely requiring less medications and services. The study by Huang and colleagues[24] only reported on 20 patients who had no readmissions or complications. Lovald and colleagues[25] recorded readmissions but not ED or office visits. Because the authors have seen that outpatient TKAs can result in more readmissions and ED/office visits, it is unlikely this has been factored into these

studies and unclear how much of an impact this will make on overall cost. Springer and colleagues[10] noted that the implementation of the Patient Care and Affordability Act has increased scrutiny of 30-day hospital readmissions. This includes the potential for 3% penalties of total hospital reimbursements. Clement and colleagues[29] estimated that if Medicare stopped reimbursing for readmissions after THA, their hospital would lose $11,494 per episode of care. Based on the available data, outpatient TKA seems to be higher risk financially when taking the fiscal consequences into consideration and more research is needed to weigh the cost saving benefits against potential implications.

SUMMARY

Outpatient total joint replacement seems safe and feasible in certain populations. From the data available, it is evident that younger patients with a lower BMI and fewer comorbidities are appropriate candidates. Many participants self-selected their outpatient status, thus more randomized trials are needed to eliminate this bias. Standardized clinical protocols and a multidisciplinary approach are vital to the success of the outpatient pathway. Larger-scale prospective randomized trials are also needed to determine how postoperative outcomes compare with a standard inpatient and who will benefit most from this intervention. Outpatient TKA has a slightly higher rate of readmission and ED visits, compared with outpatient THA. Outpatient TJA has been shown consistently cost saving; however, if hospitals are penalized for readmissions, costs may increase. PROs, when used, tend to show statistically significant improvements after outpatient joint replacement but these should be used routinely and compared with a control group in the future for maximal benefit.

REFERENCES

1. Kurtz S, Ong K, Lau E, et al. Projections of primary and revision hip and knee arthroplasty in the United States from 2005 to 2030. J Bone Joint Surg Am 2007;89(4):780.
2. Schairer WW, Sing DC, Vail TP, et al. Causes and frequency of unplanned hospital readmission after total hip arthroplasty. Clin Orthop Relat Res 2014; 472(2):464–70.
3. Ramkumar PN, Chu CT, Harris JD, et al. Causes and rates of unplanned readmissions after elective primary total joint arthroplasty: a systematic review and meta-analysis. Am J Orthop (Belle Mead NJ) 2015;44(9):397–405.

4. Ong KL, Kurtz SM, Lau E, et al. Prosthetic joint infection risk after total hip arthroplasty in the Medicare population. J Arthroplasty 2009;24(6): 105–9.

5. Whitehouse JD. The Impact of surgical site infections following orthopaedic surgery at a community hospital and a university hospital adverse quality of life, excess length of stay, and extra cost. Infect Control Hosp Epidemiol 2002;23(4):183–9.

6. Kolisek FR, McGrath MS, Jessup NM, et al. Comparison of outpatient versus inpatient total knee arthroplasty. Clin Orthop Relat Res 2009;467(6): 1438.

7. Den Hartog YM, Mathijssen NM, Vehmeijer SB. Reduced length of hospital stay after the introduction of a rapid recovery protocol for primary THA procedures. Acta Orthop 2013;84(5):444–7.

8. Goyal N, Chen AF, Padgett SE, et al. Otto Aufranc Award: a multicenter, randomized study of outpatient versus inpatient total hip arthroplasty. Clin Orthop Relat Res 2017;475(2):364–72.

9. Aynardi M, Post Z, Ong A, et al. Outpatient surgery as a means of cost reduction in total hip arthroplasty: a case-control study. HHS J 2014;10(3): 252–5.

10. Springer BD, Odum SM, Vegari DN, et al. Impact of inpatient versus outpatient total joint arthroplasty on 30-day readmission rates and unplanned episodes of care. Orthop Clin North Am 2017;48:15–23.

11. Bertin KC. Minimally invasive outpatient total hip arthroplasty. Clin Orthop Relat Res 2005;435: 154–63.

12. Dorr LD, Thomas DJ, Zu J, et al. Outpatient total hip arthroplasty. J Arthroplasty 2010;25(4):501–6.

13. Berger RA, Sanders SA, Thill ES, et al. Newer anesthesia and rehabilitation protocols enable outpatient hip replacement in selected patients. Clin Orthop Relat Res 2009;467(6):1424–30.

14. Berger RA, Jacobs JJ, Meneghini RM, et al. Rapid rehabilitation and recovery with minimally invasive total hip arthroplasty. Clin Orthop Relat Res 2004; 429:239–47.

15. Berger RA. Total hip arthroplasty using the minimally invasive two-incision approach. Clin Orthop Relat Res 2003;417:232–41.

16. Den Hartog YM, Mathijssen NM, Vehmeijer SBW. Total hip arthroplasty in an outpatient setting in 27 selected patients. Acta Orthop 2015;86(6): 667–70.

17. Winther SD, Foss OA, Wik TS, et al. 1-Year follow-up of 920 hip and knee arthroplasty patients after implementing fast-track. Acta Orthop 2015;86(1):78–85.

18. Bal BS, Lowe JA. Muscle damage in minimally invasive total hip arthroplasty: MRI evidence that it is not significant. Instr Course Lect 2008;57:223–9.

19. Woolson ST, Pouliot MA, Huddleston JI. Primary total hip arthroplasty using an anterior approach and a fracture table: short-term results from a community hospital. J Arthroplasty 2009;24(7): 999–1005.

20. Seng BE, Berend KR, Ajluni AF, et al. Anterior-supine minimally invasive total hip arthroplasty: defining the learning curve. Orthop Clin North Am 2009;40(3):343–50.

21. Phillips CB, Barrett JA, Losina E, et al. Incidence rates of dislocation, pulmonary embolism, and deep infection during the first six months after elective total hip replacement. J Bone Joint Surg Am 2003;85(1):20–6.

22. Kesterke N, Egeter J, Erhardt JB, et al. Patient-reported outcome assessment after total joint replacement: comparison of questionnaire completion times on paper and tablet computer. Arch Orthop Trauma Surg 2015;135:935–41.

23. Specht K, Kjaersgaard-Anderson P, Pederson BD. Patient experience in fast-track hip and knee arthroplasty – a qualitative study. J Clin Nurs 2015;25:836–45.

24. Huang A, Ryu JJ, Dervin G. Cost savings of outpatient versus standard inpatient total knee arthroplasty. Can J Surg 2016;60(1):57–62.

25. Lovald ST, Ong KL, Malkani AL, et al. Complications, mortality and costs for outpatients and short-stay total knee arthroplasty patients in comparison to standard-stay patients. J Arthroplasty 2014;29(3):510–5.

26. Berger RA, Kusuma SK, Sanders SA, et al. The feasibility and perioperative complications of outpatient knee arthroplasty. Clin Orthop Relat Res 2009; 467(6):1443–9.

27. Berger RA, Sanders S, D'Ambrogio E, et al. Minimally invasive quadriceps-sparing TKA: results of a comprehensive pathway for outpatient TKA. J Knee Surg 2006;19:145–8.

28. Goble EM, Justin DF. Minimally invasive total knee replacement: principles and technique. Orthop Clin North Am 2004;35:235.

29. Clement RC, Derman PB, Graham DS, et al. Risk factors, causes, and the economic implications of unplanned readmissions following total hip arthroplasty. J Arthroplasty 2013;28(8 Suppl):7–10.

Trauma

The Role of Implant Removal in Orthopedic Trauma

Eric A. Barcak, DO*, Michael J. Beebe, MD,
John C. Weinlein, MD

KEYWORDS

• Implant removal • Orthopedic implants • Retained implant • Painful implant

KEY POINTS

• Implant removal is a common procedure performed after orthopedic trauma.
• Indications for implant removal with the goal of decreasing pain and/or increasing function are controversial.
• Implants are routinely removed from the ankle syndesmosis and midfoot (Lisfranc injuries), although there are few supportive data.
• Complications are not uncommon with implant removal.

INTRODUCTION

"You never look good taking out hardware" is a phrase commonly uttered by surgeons when removing orthopedic implants after trauma. Although many implant removal procedures are completed in a timely manner without complications, others are fraught with frustration, broken implants, altered anatomy, and unfamiliar situations. These issues raise the question, when is implant removal indicated? Surgeons remove implants for many reasons, including failure, malposition, infection, cosmesis, and pain. In addition, planned implant removal often is done when joints, such as the ankle syndesmosis and the midfoot, are spanned. Although there is general agreement on the indications for implant removal, such as failure, malposition (eg, intraarticular implant), or infection, the indications for implant removal with the goals of decreasing pain or improving function are controversial. The article discusses the current role of implant removal in orthopedic trauma.

GENERAL

There are no specific guidelines regarding orthopedic implant removal after trauma. Often, removal is offered to patients when no other reasonable explanation is apparent for their pain. Surgeons are frequently left telling these patients that implant removal may or may not help with symptoms. This situation can be discouraging for both patients and surgeons. Several studies have attempted to quantify patient benefits and costs of such procedures,[1–7] but no definitive indications have been established.

To evaluate implant removal from a patient's perspective, Reith and colleagues[6] surveyed 332 subjects who had elective implant removal after fracture union. Indications for removal included pain (31%); decreased function (31%); and, interestingly, surgeon recommendation (68%). Implants were removed from both upper and lower extremities, as well as the pelvis (2%) and spine (2%). Implant removal after ankle surgery was the most common (21%). After implant removal, 96% of the subjects had decreased

Department of Orthopaedic Surgery, University of Tennessee-Campbell Clinic, Regional One Health, Memphis, TN, USA
* Corresponding author. Campbell Clinic 1211 Union Avenue #500 Memphis, TN 38104.
E-mail address: ericbarcak@gmail.com

Orthop Clin N Am 49 (2018) 45–53
https://doi.org/10.1016/j.ocl.2017.08.014
0030-5898/18/© 2017 Elsevier Inc. All rights reserved.

pain and 72% demonstrated improved function. A 10% complication rate was associated with implant removal, with wound complications being the most common (36%). Other common complications included infection (21%), nerve injury (14%), and incomplete implant removal (12%). Despite these findings, 66% of subjects who had complications stated they would undergo implant removal again.

Minkowitz and colleagues[4] evaluated 60 subjects with united fractures that had been treated with internal fixation, all of whom complained of continued pain in the region near the implants after fracture healing. Baseline subjective functional outcome measures were obtained before implant removal. Of the 57 subjects who completed follow-up, 50 had implant removal from the lower extremity, most commonly from the ankle (22 subjects). Few had implant removal from the olecranon (3), forearm (1), or clavicle (0). At 1-year follow-up, all subjects were satisfied and stated they would have the procedure again. Significant improvements were seen in functional measures (Short Musculoskeletal Functional Assessment [SMFA] and Short Form Health Survey [SF]-36 physical component) and pain (visual analog scale [VAS]), and 53% of subjects had complete resolution of pain. Remarkably, no complications were reported with any of the surgeries.

Although pain and functional improvements are important factors in determining the need for implant removal, cost also needs to be considered. In a 2011 study from Nigeria, Onche and colleagues[5] concluded that routine removal of orthopedic implants after fracture healing was a "great waste of highly needed cash." In their subjects, the mean hospital stay was 2.6 days with a mean cost of $708 per subject. Mean time missed from school or work was around 16 days. Although it is difficult to compare costs between this study and health care in other countries, cost remains an important factor in elective surgical decision-making. Other studies have reported similar periods of missed work associated with implant removal (11–14 days).[1,7]

Although these studies are important, all have limitations. They are all composed of heterogeneous groups of subjects with different injuries treated with different implants. Other studies have discussed the benefits and complications associated with implant removal in specific regions of the body.

MIDFOOT OR LISFRANC JOINT

Opinions about planned implant removal in Lisfranc injuries vary widely among surgeons. Traditionally, dislocations of the tarsometatarsal joints have been treated with screw fixation when metatarsal base comminution is absent. Even without a formal fusion, there is little evidence for the need to remove transarticular screws from the Lisfranc joint because it is a nonessential joint of the foot: unlike the fourth and fifth tarsometatarsal joints, the intercuneiform joints and first through third tarsometatarsal have very little physiologic motion and, thus, transarticular implants do not significantly alter normal foot mechanics.[8,9] Because of the frequency of screw breakage, however, many surgeons routinely remove these screws, generally at around 4 months after injury.[10,11]

More recently, plate fixation has been used to avoid injury to chondral surfaces from transarticular screw fixation.[11–13] Although plate fixation of Lisfranc injuries is not a new concept and has been shown to be biomechanically similar to screw fixation, the advent of thinner locking and nonlocking minifragment plates, as well as custom midfoot plates, has expanded the role of plate fixation.[12] There is little evidence to support or refute the routine removal of plate fixation; however, because the implants are not transarticular, broken screws or plates, even if left in place, are less likely to be a concern.[11] Nonetheless, some surgeons still recommend routine removal.[14]

Several recent studies have focused on fixation techniques that do not require implant removal. Suture-button devices have long been used in other injuries, but their use in Lisfranc injuries is becoming more common.[15,16] In a cadaver study, Panchbhavi and colleagues[16] found no significant difference in displacement between suture-button fixation and screw fixation, whereas Ahmed and colleagues[15] found significantly more motion at the joint with suture-button fixation, but this was equal to the physiologic motion at the Lisfranc joint under similar loading. Unless there is a wound complication, use of a suture-button essentially negates the need for removal; however, suture-button fixation has been reserved for only low-energy injuries. Other fixation options, such as polylactic acid screws, have been used by some surgeons, but the evidence for their clinical use is still limited and they are not currently mainstream.[13,17]

The more permanent option of fusion can help to significantly decrease the rate of implant removal[18] while potentially improving outcomes, at least in primarily ligamentous injuries.[9] In a meta-analysis, Smith and colleagues[19] found that the risk of implant removal after primary arthrodesis was significantly less than that after open reduction and internal fixation; however, they also found no significant difference in patient-reported outcomes between fusion and open reduction and internal fixation (ORIF).

In summary, although the rate of implant removal in Lisfranc injuries is high, the frequency of removal is artificially elevated because many surgeons routinely schedule removal when there is little to no evidence to support the need.

SYNDESMOSIS OR FIBULAR INJURIES

The treatment of injuries involving the ankle syndesmosis continues to be among the most studied topics in orthopedic trauma. Despite recent advances in fixation techniques, the gold standard for treatment is still considered to be a stainless steel screw.[20] Although a screw may provide the rigidity necessary for healing, it also may create an environment that does not allow the inherent physiologic motion of the distal tibiofibular joint.[21] Some investigators have argued that the presence of this screw is a potential pain generator and, once ligamentous healing has occurred, screw removal is necessary to allow appropriate motion.[21] A counterargument is that screw removal leads to the potential for early displacement and is associated with increased cost and risk of surgical complications. Studies have provided mixed results regarding syndesmotic screw status and functional outcomes. Tucker and colleagues[22] evaluated the functional outcomes of 63 subjects with syndesmotic injuries, 43 of whom had screw removal and 20 who had screws left in place. Those with retained screws scored higher on the Olerud-Molander Ankle Score (OMAS) and experienced less pain than those with screw removal. The investigators advocated screws being left in situ, with removal in symptomatic subjects only. Boyle and colleagues[23] reported a randomized controlled trial of 51 subjects who had syndesmosis screw fixation of ankle fractures. Subjects were randomized to either screw removal at 3 months or screw retention. At 1 year, no difference was found between the groups in functional outcomes (OMAS and American Orthopedic Foot and Ankle Society Score), ankle range of motion (ROM), pain, and radiographic reduction. Of note, 76% of the subjects with retained screws had implant failure or loosening at final follow-up.

In a comprehensive literature review,[24] 7 studies evaluating outcomes and syndesmotic screw status were analyzed. No significant difference in functional outcomes was seen between retained or removed screws. Interestingly, screws that were either loose or broken seemed to have similar or improved outcomes compared with subjects who had screws removed. One study[25] demonstrated lower functional outcome measures with intact retained screws, and the investigators concluded that subjects with loose or broken screws are unlikely to benefit from screw removal. In a retrospective study of 82 subjects with a minimum of 1-year follow-up,[20] clinical outcomes were similar in subjects with screw retention and subjects with screw removal; however, subjects with broken screws had the best clinical outcomes. A more recent systematic review[26] that included 2 randomized controlled trials and 9 case-control studies concluded that, although there are many shortcomings listed in the current literature, routine syndesmotic screw removal is not supported.

Malreduction of the syndesmosis has been cited in multiple studies as a common problem associated with surgery. Song and colleagues[27] evaluated bilateral postoperative ankle computed tomography (CT) scans to evaluate reductions in 25 subjects with syndesmosis injuries treated with screw fixation; 9 (36%) had malreductions. All syndesmosis screws were removed at 3 months after surgery and a second CT scan was obtained to evaluate any changes; 8 of the 9 malreductions showed appropriate reduction of the joint after screw removal. Moreover, there were no reported cases of loss of reduction. No functional outcome measurements were performed in this study.

Removal of syndesmosis screws is not without complications. Schepers and colleagues[28] reported a 22.4% complication rate associated with screw removal in 76 subjects. Complications included wound infection (9.2%) and recurrent diastasis (6.6%). Andersen and colleagues[29] evaluated 106 subjects who had syndesmosis screw removal and found a 5% percent infection rate, with serious infection requiring hospitalization in 2% of the subjects.

Ultimately, it is up to the treating surgeon to discuss risks and benefits of screw removal with the patient. Although the current data concerning functional outcomes are not entirely clear, they do demonstrate that implant failure and loosening are common with retained screws and this possibility should be discussed with the patient before surgery. Additionally, patients with intact screws and associated ankle pain may benefit from removal more than patients who have loose or broken implants. Patients with a malreduced syndesmosis also may benefit from screw removal.

Syndesmotic screws are not the only implant around the ankle that is commonly removed. Patients with surgically treated ankle fractures often have lateral pain over plate and screw constructs. Brown and colleagues[30] reported a 31% incidence of lateral pain after operative treatment of 126 unstable ankle fractures. Subjects with lateral ankle pain had lower functional scores (SMFA and SF-36) than patients without lateral ankle pain. Of the 29 subjects who elected or desired implant removal, only 11 of 22 with removal had improvement. No significant differences were reported in functional outcomes aforementioned between those who did and did not undergo implant removal. Differing from the aforementioned study, Jacobsen and colleagues[31] reported improvement in approximately 75% of subjects after removal of implants used for ankle fracture fixation.

TIBIAL PLATEAU FRACTURES

Tibia plateau fractures can be devastating injuries from a functional standpoint. Restoration of joint stability and mechanical axis, as well as meniscal repair, have been associated with improved outcomes. Lateral, and sometimes medial, plating techniques are generally used for ORIF. Garner and colleagues[32] compared functional outcomes at 12-month follow-up in 2 groups of subjects with united tibial plateau fractures that had been treated with ORIF. One group (39 subjects) had elective implant removal, whereas the second group (36 subjects) retained their implants. Significantly better clinical outcomes were found in the group who had their implants removed. Interestingly, no significant differences in pain (VAS) were identified between cohorts. The investigators suggested that patients who are dissatisfied with outcomes after tibial plateau surgery can be offered implant removal to help improve function; however, pain improvement may not occur.

PATELLAR FRACTURES

The anterior knee can be an especially troubling region for implants because of the limited soft tissue that surrounds the bony structures. As a result, prominent or symptomatic implants are a commonly reported complication associated with patellar fixation. LeBrun and colleagues[33] reported that, in 27 subjects with isolated patellar fractures treated with ORIF, 14 (52%) had required implant removal because of symptoms at an average 6-year follow-up. Five of 13 subjects who had retained implants complained

of implant-related pain. Lazaro and colleagues[34] evaluated functional impairment in a cohort of 30 subjects with patellar fractures treated with ORIF. As in the study by LeBrun and colleagues,[33] symptomatic implants were common and required removal in 37% of the subjects. Additionally, anterior knee pain during activities of daily living was reported by 24 (80%) of the 30 subjects.

Tension band constructs continue to be the mainstay of treatment of most patellar fractures. Traditional use of Kirschner wires resulted in high rates of implant removal.[35] More recently, the use of suture and cannulated screws for tension band constructs has gained popularity. Hoshino and colleagues[36] retrospectively compared complications in subjects with patellar fractures treated with either Kirschner wires (315 subjects) or cannulated screws (133 subjects). Most tension band constructs were completed with 18-gauge wire. A significant difference ($P = .003$) was found between the groups regarding elective implant removal, with 37% of the subjects in Kirschner wire group having implant removal compared with 23% in the cannulated screw group. Overall, maintenance of fixation was similar between the 2 groups. The investigators did not discuss if implant removal improved pain or functional status.

TIBIAL AND FEMORAL SHAFT FRACTURES

Intramedullary nailing (IMN) is the gold standard for treatment of lower extremity long-bone fractures. Although predictable healing usually occurs with this treatment modality, some patients continue to have pain associated with their injury. Pain may be secondary to proximal or distal interlocking screws. Alternatively, some investigators have attributed this pain to modulus mismatch between the metal of the intramedullary nail and the host bone. Anterior knee pain also is a common complaint after IMN of the tibia. Similar to other areas of the body, there are no clear guidelines about removal of these implants.

A recent prospective study reported on 57 subjects with tibial shaft fractures treated with IMN, 24 of whom had moderate to severe postoperative knee pain. Removal of the IMN significantly relieved pain in 18 and made no change in pain levels in 6. Subjects with tibial nails within 10 mm of the tibial plateau were more likely to have pain.[37] Another study evaluated outcomes of 43 subjects who had elective tibial nail removal, most commonly because of anterior knee pain (48%).[38] Overall, 72% of subjects were satisfied after their surgery. Complications occurred in 12 subjects (13%); superficial infection was the most common (6%). Of the 48 subjects in whom nail removal was indicated, the nails could not be removed in 5. Dodenhoff and colleagues[39] reported that 33 (41%) of 80 subjects with femoral shaft fractures treated with IMN had persistent thigh pain after union. Of these, 21 (64%) had heterotopic ossification and 3 (9%) had prominent interlocking screws, but 4 (12%) had no observed radiographic abnormality. Seventeen subjects had nail removal because of pain; however, only 11 (65%) reported improvement. Better outcomes were reported by Bednar and colleagues[40] in 20 subjects who had implant-related pain after union of femoral shaft fractures: 17 (85%) had pain relief after intramedullary nail removal. Two large studies reported low rates of refracture with nail removal after union of femoral shaft fractures; only 1 refracture in 234 nail removals.[41,42]

HIP AND PELVIS

Shortening of the femoral neck is common with internal fixation of femoral neck fractures; many implants are designed to allow shortening. This shortening often results in prominent implants around the trochanteric region. Zielinski and colleagues[43] compared functional outcomes after removal of fracture fixation devices about the hip in 22 subjects with outcomes in a matched cohort of 22 subjects with retained implants. Significant improvement in functional outcome scores (SF-12 and Western Ontario and McMaster Universities Osteoarthritis Index [WOMAC]) was seen after implant removal compared with the control group with retained implants. Complications occurred in 8 (22%) subjects with implant removal, but recurrent fracture did not occur. Of note, final follow-up for some subjects was less than 6 months. Although not reported in the study by Zielinski and colleagues,[43] fracture or refracture of the femoral neck should be considered a risk of implant removal about the hip. Yoon and colleagues[44] reported 6 (9%) femoral neck fractures after compression hip screw removal in 67 united intertrochanteric femoral fractures. All fractures occurred within 1 month of implant removal. Recently, Quade and colleagues[45] reported the potential benefits of iliosacral or transsacral screw removal after operative treatment of posterior pelvic ring injuries. The investigators identified 471 subjects treated over 10 years with iliosacral or transsacral screws, 25 (5.4%) of whom had screws

removed at a mean of 10.7 months after pelvic injury. Of the 18 subjects for whom outcomes were available, 15 (83%) reported improvement in pain.

OLECRANON

Like many injuries, fractures about the olecranon vary widely in complexity and instability. As such, the treatment options also cross a broad spectrum. The most traditional approach to fixation involves the tension band technique, a construct traditionally consisting of 2 longitudinal Kirschner wires with a flexible wire looped around the Kirschner wires and placed through a drill hole in the stable segment of the distal ulna. Huang and colleagues[46] retrospectively reviewed 78 displaced olecranon fractures treated with tension band constructs and evaluated placement of the distal aspect of the Kirschner wire in 3 locations: in the proximal ulnar canal, through the anterior ulnar cortex, and in the distal ulnar canal. They found that wires placed intramedullary into only the proximal canal had a higher risk of proximal pin migration and elbow irritation compared with longer, more distally reaching wires or wires penetrating the anterior cortex. Eight (33.3%) of 24 subjects with proximal intramedullary wires requested implant removal, compared with 3 (10.7%) of 28 with bicortical wires, and 2 (7.7%) of 26 with distal intramedullary wires. There was no difference in healing rate or other complications. Contrary to this finding, Chalidis and colleagues[47] retrospectively reviewed 62 subjects treated with tension band wiring of the olecranon and found that there was no difference in the rate of pin loosening or migration between anterior cortex perforation and short intramedullary placement. They did find, however, that 82.3% of subjects had implant removal and two-thirds of those subjects still complained of mild pain during daily activities. Similarly, Chan and Donnelly[48] reviewed 63 subjects with either intramedullary or bicortical wire placement and found no difference in the rate of removal (19% vs 25% respectively, $P = .89$). Their rate of removal was, however, significantly lower than that reported by Chalidis and colleagues.[47]

Although locked plate fixation of the olecranon is well-accepted for repair of comminuted fracture patterns, an increasing number of surgeons have turned to anatomic precontoured plate fixation of even simple transverse olecranon fractures. Schliemann and colleagues[49] compared tension band fixation to locking compression plate fixation in 26 displaced, noncomminuted olecranon fractures, 13 with a precontoured locking compression plate and 13 with tension band wiring. At a mean follow-up of 43 months, the mean Disability of the Arm, Shoulder, and Hand (DASH) score was 14 points in the compression plate group and 12.5 points in tension band group. Twelve (92%) of the 13 subjects in the compression plate group achieved good-to-excellent results on the Mayo Elbow Performance score compared with 10 (77%) of 13 in the tension band group. There were no significant differences between the 2 groups regarding the objective clinical and subjective radiographic outcomes. Implant-related irritation requiring implant removal occurred more frequently in the tension band group (12 of 13) than in the compression plate group (7 of 13).

Less common techniques have been used with the goal of minimizing soft-tissue irritation while still providing stable fixation. Although the technique has been more commonly used for fixation of olecranon osteotomies, the use of a large intramedullary screw with a washer may provide more stable fixation than a tension band, while limiting the risk of soft-tissue irritation.[50,51] More novel devices, including multiplanar locked intramedullary nails, may offer similar advantages in more comminuted patterns, but the results and availability of implants currently are quite limited.[52–54]

Overall, the rate of olecranon implant removal varies widely among studies and centers, but is often quite high. The rate of tension band removal ranges from 11% to 92%,[47,55–58] whereas the rate of plate removal ranges from 0% to 54%.[55,59–61]

CLAVICULAR FRACTURES

Clavicular fractures are among the most commonly treated fractures by orthopedic surgeons. Although specific operative criteria continue to evolve, the need for implant removal remains a constant concern.[62–64] The limited soft tissue surrounding the clavicle, especially in thin patients, makes plate prominence a concern from a cosmetic standpoint and can be bothersome while wearing specific items, such as backpacks. Although plate removal for a failed or infected implant is usually necessary, its effect on functional outcomes and pain is more difficult to determine. Naimark and colleagues[65] found that subjects with implant removal reported worse shoulder function than those who had retained implants. Moreover, there is concern

that plate removal could potentially result in refracture. In a systematic review of complications associated with plate fixation of clavicular fractures, Wijdicks and colleagues[66] analyzed 11 studies and found that plate irritation was commonly reported (9% to 64%). Of note, studies with higher rates of plate irritation used noncontoured plates. Additionally, the investigators found a relatively small risk of refracture after implant removal (1% to 5%). Wang and colleagues[7] evaluated 48 subjects at an average follow-up of 13 months to determine if plate removal is necessary after clavicular fracture union. Twenty-seven subjects had plates removed, whereas 21 retained their implants. Implant removal occurred for many reasons, including pain (6), limited ROM during sports (13), interferences with daily activities (10), and concerns about refracture (3). Overall, 96% of subjects who had implant removal were satisfied with their results, as were 86% of subjects with plate retention. Of the latter group, 71% complained of local pain and prominence but stated that the discomfort did not significantly interfere with their quality of life. There was no significant difference in shoulder function between the 2 groups. The investigators concluded that plate irritation is common (88%) after fixation of clavicular fractures, especially in young patients who are active, but they did not recommend routine plate removal after fracture union.

SUMMARY

Although implant removal is common after fracture healing, especially from the ankle syndesmosis, removal may not decrease pain or increase function. There are few data in the literature to allow evidence-based decision-making. The risk of complications from implant removal must be weighed against the possible benefits and the likelihood of improving the patient's symptoms.

REFERENCES

1. Boerger TO, Patel G, Murphy JP. Is routine removal of intramedullary nails justified. Injury 1999;30:79–81.
2. Böstman O, Pihlajamäki H. Routine implant removal after fracture surgery: a potentially reducible consumer of hospital resources in trauma units. J Trauma 1996;41:846–9.
3. Busam ML, Esther RJ, Obremskey WT. Hardware removal: indications and expectations. J Am Acad Orthop Surg 2006;14:113–20.
4. Minkowitz R, Bhadsavle S, Walsh M, et al. Removal of painful orthopaedic implants after fracture union. J Bone Joint Surg Am 2007;89:1906–12.

5. Onche II, Osagie OE, INuhu S. Removal of orthopaedic implants: indications, outcome and economic implications. J West Afr Coll Surg 2011;1:101–12.

6. Reith G, Schmitz-Greven V, Hensel KO, et al. Metal implant removal: benefits and drawbacks—a patient survey. BMC Surg 2015;15:96.

7. Wang J, Chidambaram R, Mok D. Is removal of clavicle plate after fracture union necessary? Int J Shoulder Surg 2011;5:85–9.

8. Bernischke SK, Meinberg E, Anderson SA, et al. Fractures and dislocations of the midfoot: Lisfranc and Chopart injuries. J Bone Joint Surg Am 2012;94:1326–37.

9. Ly TV, Coetzee JC. Treatment of primarily ligamentous Lisfranc joint injuries: primary arthrodesis compared with open reduction and internal fixation. A prospective randomized study. J Bone Joint Surg Am 2006;88:514–20.

10. Dubois-Ferriere V, Lübbeke A, Chowdhary A, et al. Clinical outcomes and development of symptomatic osteoarthritis 2 to 24 years after surgical treatment of tarsometatarsal joint complex injuries. J Bone Joint Surg Am 2016;98:713–20.

11. Watson TS, Shurnas PS, Denker J. Treatment of Lisfranc joint injury: current concepts. J Am Acad Orthop Surg 2010;18:718–28.

12. Alberta FG, Aronow MS, Barrero M, et al. Ligamentous Lisfranc joint injuries: a biomechanical comparison of dorsal plate and transarticular screw fixation. Foot Ankle Int 2005;26:462–73.

13. Thordarson DB, Hurvitz G. PLA screw fixation of Lisfranc injuries. Foot Ankle Int 2002;23:1003–7.

14. Van Koperen PJ, de Jong VM, Luitse JS, et al. Functional outcomes after temporary bridging with locking plates in Lisfranc injuries. J Foot Ankle Surg 2016;55:922–6.

15. Ahmed S, Bolt B, McBryde A. Comparison of standard screw fixation versus suture button fixation in Lisfranc ligament injuries. Foot Ankle Int 2010;31:892–6.

16. Panchbhavi VK, Vallurupalli S, Yang J, et al. Screw fixation compared with suture-button fixation of isolated Lisfranc ligament injuries. J Bone Joint Surg Am 2009;91:1143–8.

17. Ahmad J, Jones K. Randomized, prospective comparison of bioabsorbable and steel screw fixation of Lisfranc injuries. J Orthop Trauma 2016;30:676–81.

18. Henning JA, Jones CB, Sietsema DL, et al. Open reduction internal fixation versus primary arthrodesis for Lisfranc injuries: a prospective randomized study. Foot Ankle Int 2009;30:913–22.

19. Smith N, Stone C, Furey A. Does open reduction and internal fixation versus primary arthrodesis improve patient outcomes for Lisfranc trauma? a systematic review and meta-analysis. Clin Orthop Relat Res 2016;474:1445–52.

20. Kaftandziev I, Spasov M, Trpeski S, et al. Fate of the syndesmotic screw—search for a prudent solution. Injury 2015;46(Suppl 6):S125–9.

21. Miller AN, Paul O, Boraiah S, et al. Functional outcomes after syndesmotic screw fixation and removal. J Orthop Trauma 2010;24:12–6.

22. Tucker A, Street J, Kealey D, et al. Functional outcomes following syndesmotic fixation: a comparison of screws retained in situ versus routine removal—is it really necessary? Injury 2013;44:1880–4.

23. Boyle MJ, Gao R, Frampton CM, et al. Removal of the syndesmotic screw after the surgical treatment of the ankle in adult patients does not affect one-year outcomes: a randomized controlled trial. Bone Joint J 2014;96-B:1699–705.

24. Schepers T. To retain or remove the syndesmotic screw: a review of literature. Arch Orthop Trauma Surg 2011;131:879–83.

25. Manjoo A, Sanders DW, Tieszer C, et al. Functional and radiographic results of patients with syndesmotic screw fixation: implications for screw removal. J Orthop Trauma 2010;24:2–8.

26. Dingemans SA, Rammelt S, White TO, et al. Should syndesmotic screws be removed after surgical fixation of unstable fractures? a systematic review. Bone Joint J 2016;98-B:1497–504.

27. Song DJ, Lanzi JT, Groth AT, et al. The effect of syndesmosis screw removal on the reduction of the distal tibiofibular joint. A prospective radiographic study. Foot Ankle Int 2014;35:543–8.

28. Schepers T, Van Lieshout EM, de Vries MR, et al. Complications of syndesmotic screw removal. Foot Ankle Int 2011;32:1040–4.

29. Andersen MR, Frihagen F, Madsen JE, et al. High complication rate after syndesmotic screw removal. Injury 2015;46:2283–7.

30. Brown OL, Dirschl DR, Obremskey WT. Incidence of hardware-related pain and its effect on functional outcomes after open reduction and internal fixation of ankle fractures. J Orthop Trauma 2001;15:271–4.

31. Jacobsen S, Honnens de Lichtenberg M, Jensen CM, et al. Removal of internal fixation—the effect on patients' complaints: a study of 66 cases of removal of internal fixation after malleolar fractures. Foot Ankle Int 1994;15:170–1.

32. Garner MR, Thacher RR, Ni A, et al. Elective removal of implants after open reduction and internal fixation of tibial plateau fractures improves clinical outcomes. Arch Orthop Trauma Surg 2015;135:1491–6.

33. LeBrun CT, Langford JR, Sagi HC. Functional outcomes after operatively treated patella fractures. J Orthop Trauma 2012;26:422–6.

34. Lazaro LE, Wellman DS, Sauro G, et al. Outcomes after operative fixation of complete articular

patellar fractures: assessment of functional impairment. J Bone Joint Surg 2013;95:e96(1-8).

35. Kumar G, Mereddy PK, Hakkalamani S, et al. Implant removal following surgical stabilization of patella fracture. Orthopedics 2010;33(5).

36. Hoshino CM, Tran W, Tiberi JV, et al. Complications following tension-band fixation of patellar fractures with cannulated screws compared with Kirschner wires. J Bone Joint Surg Am 2013;95: 653–9.

37. Zhang S, Wu X, Liu L, et al. Removal of interlocking intramedullary nail for relieve of knee pain after tibial fracture repair. A prospective study. J Orthop Surg (Hong Kong) 2017;25(1). 2309499016684748.

38. Pathak SK, Maheshwari P, Prashanthraj M, et al. Intramedullary nails: should it be removed after fracture healing? Int Surg J 2016;3:1603–5.

39. Dodenhoff RM, Dainton JN, Hutchins PM. Proximal thigh pain after femoral nailing. J Bone Joint Surg Br 1997;79-B:738–41.

40. Bednar DA, Ali P. Intramedullary nailing of femoral shaft fractures: reoperation and return to work. Can J Surg 1993;36:464–6.

41. Brumback RJ, Ellison TS, Poka A, et al. Intramedullary nailing of femoral shaft fractures. Part III: long-term effects of static interlocking fixation. J Bone Joint Surg Am 1992;74:106–12.

42. Wolinsky PR, McCarty E, Shyr Y, et al. Reamed intramedullary nailing of the femur: 551 cases. J Trauma 1999;46:392–9.

43. Zielinski SM, Heetveld MJ, Bhandari M, et al. Implant removal after internal fixation of a femoral neck fracture: effects on physical functioning. J Orthop Trauma 2015;29:e285–92.

44. Yoon PW, Kwon JE, Yoo JJ, et al. Femoral neck fracture after removal of the compression hip screw from healed intertrochanteric fractures. J Orthop Trauma 2013;27:696–701.

45. Quade J, Beebe M, Auston D, et al. Symptomatic ilio-sacral screw removal following pelvic trauma. Paper 440, presented at American Academy of Orthopaedic Surgeons. San Diego (CA), March 15, 2017. Available at: https://www.aaos.org/uploadedFiles/2017%20Final%20Program_compressed.pdf. Accessed July 14, 2017.

46. Huang TW, Wu CC, Fan FK, et al. Tension band wiring for olecranon fractures: relative stability of Kirschner wires in various configurations. J Trauma 2010;68:173–6.

47. Chalidis BE, Sachinis NC, Samoladas EP, et al. Is tension band wiring technique the "gold standard" for the treatment of olecranon fractures? a long term functional study. J Orthop Surg Res 2008;3:9.

48. Chan KW, Donnelly KJ. Does K-wire position in tension band wiring of olecranon fractures affect its complications and removal of metal rate? J Orthop 2014;12:111–7.

49. Schliemann B, Raschke MJ, Groene P, et al. Comparison of tension band wiring and precontoured locking compression plate fixation in mayo type IIA olecranon fractures. Acta Orthop Belg 2014; 80:106–11.

50. Hutchinson DT, Horwitz DS, Ha G, et al. Cyclic loading of olecranon fracture fixation constructs. J Bone Joint Surg 2003;85:831–7.

51. Argintar E, Cohen M, Egiseder A, et al. Clinical results of olecranon fractures treated with multiplanar locked intramedullary nailing. J Orthop Trauma 2013;27:140–4.

52. Woods BI, Rosario BL, Siska PA, et al. Determining the efficacy of screw and washer fixation as a method for securing olecranon osteotomies used in the surgical management of intraarticular distal humerus fractures. J Orthop Trauma 2015; 29:44–9.

53. Edwards SG, Argintar E, Lamb J. Management of comminuted proximal ulna fracture-dislocations using a multiplanar locking intramedullary nail. Tech Hand Up Extrem Surg 2011;15:106–14.

54. Nowak TE, Burkhart KJ, Mueller LP, et al. New intramedullary locking nail for olecranon fracture fixation–an in vitro biomechanical comparison with tension band wiring. J Trauma 2010;69: E56–61.

55. Hume MC, Wiss DA. Olecranon fractures. A clinical and radiographic comparison of tension band wiring and plate fixation. Clin Orthop Relat Res 1992;285:229–35.

56. Macko D, Szabo RM. Complications of tension-band wiring of olecranon fractures. J Bone Joint Surg Am 1985;67:1396–401.

57. Murphy DF, Greene WB, Dameron TB. Displaced olecranon fractures in adults. Clinical evaluation. Clin Orthop Relat Res 1987;224:215–23.

58. Wolfgang G, Burke F, Bush D, et al. Surgical treatment of displaced olecranon fractures by tension band wiring technique. Clin Orthop Relat Res 1987;224:192–204.

59. Bailey CS, MacDermid J, Patterson SD, et al. Outcome of plate fixation of olecranon fractures. J Orthop Trauma 2001;15:542–8.

60. Tejwani NC, Garnham IR, Wolinsky PR, et al. Posterior olecranon plating: biomechanical and clinical evaluation of a new operative technique. Bull Hosp Jt Dis 2001;61:27–31.

61. Wellman DS, Lazaro LE, Cymerman RM, et al. Treatment of olecranon fractures with 2.4- and 2.7-mm plating techniques. J Orthop Trauma 2015;29:36–43.

62. Leroux T, Wasserstein D, Henry P, et al. Rate of and risk factors for reoperations after open reduction and internal fixation of midshaft clavicle fractures:

a population-based study in Ontario, Canada. J Bone Joint Surg Am 2014;96:1119–25.

63. Schemitsch LA, Schemitsch EH, Kuzyk P, et al. Prognostic factors for reoperation after plate fixation of the midshaft clavicle. J Orthop Trauma 2015;29:533–7.

64. Shen WJ, Liu TJ, Shen YS. Plate fixation of fresh displaced midshaft clavicle fractures. Injury 1999;30: 497–500.

65. Naimark M, Dufka FL, Han R, et al. Plate fixation of midshaft clavicular fractures: patient-reported outcomes and hardware-related complications. J Shoulder Elbow Surg 2016;25:739–46.

66. Wijdicks FJ, Van der Meijden OA, Millett PJ, et al. Systematic review of the complications of plate fixation of clavicle fractures. Arch Orthop Trauma Surg 2012;132:617–25.

Pediatrics

Outpatient Pediatric Orthopedic Surgery

Daniel J. Miller, MD*, Susan E. Nelson, MD, MPH, Apurva S. Shah, MD, MBA, Theodore J. Ganley, MD, John (Jack) M. Flynn, MD

KEYWORDS

- Pediatrics orthopedic surgery • Day surgery • Ambulatory surgery • Perioperative pathways
- Regional anesthesia

KEY POINTS

- Interest in pediatric outpatient surgery as a safe and efficient alternative to inpatient perioperative management is increasing.
- Evidence suggests that in appropriately selected patients, outpatient surgery decreases costs and avoids detrimental psychological effects of hospital admission.
- Team expertise in the comprehensive perioperative management of pediatric patient and family education is essential for successful outpatient postoperative management.
- Outpatient pediatric orthopedic surgery should be considered in consultation with patients and families, in the context of appropriate patient and surgical factors.

INTRODUCTION

Outpatient surgery (also known to as ambulatory surgery, same-day surgery, or day surgery) refers to a surgical procedure that is performed without an overnight stay in a hospital.[1] As the modern health care system evolves, emphasis has been placed on delivering high-quality care in the most safe and efficient manner possible. In light of this, there has been an evolving focus on outpatient procedures in many orthopedic interventions over the past 30 years.[1,2] Although most prevalent in adult orthopedic surgery, this trend has been observed in the pediatric population as well.[3,4]

As experience with outpatient surgery increases, selection criteria has widened.[5] Outpatient surgery is an attractive option for a variety of procedures that can lead to decreased individual and societal costs compared with inpatient hospitalization while achieving equivalent health outcomes.[1] The detrimental psychosocial effects of inpatient hospitalization on children may also be mitigated by an outpatient surgery approach.

Despite the potential benefits of outpatient surgery, there are several limitations that are particularly relevant to the heterogeneous patient population one encounters in pediatric orthopedics. This review summarizes the most recent literature published on the role of pediatric outpatient orthopedic surgery, including current practice trends and outcomes. Strategies for integrating outpatient procedures into a pediatric orthopedic practice are discussed.

POTENTIAL ADVANTAGES OF OUTPATIENT SURGERY

Outpatient surgery has numerous potential benefits when compared with inpatient care. In the current health care environment, systems are increasingly focused on improving *value* delivery by decreasing the cost of treatment while

Disclosure Statement: The authors have nothing to disclose that relates to the subject matter or materials discussed in this article.

Division of Orthopaedic Surgery, Children's Hospital of Philadelphia, 2nd Floor Wood Building, 3401 Civic Center Boulevard, Philadelphia, PA 19104, USA

* Corresponding author.

E-mail address: daniel.james.miller@gmail.com

optimizing the quality of care delivered.[6] Outpatient surgery is particularly advantageous in this respect. Costs for outpatient orthopedic procedures are estimated to be 17% to 68% less than equivalent procedures with an inpatient stay.[1,5] Savings associated with outpatient procedures are attributed to lack of overnight admission charges and costs associated with inpatient care services, such as facility depreciation and maintenance, medications, nursing, and therapy services.[1]

Outpatient surgery may have particular psychological benefits for the pediatric population. Continuous support of a nurturing family is indispensable to a child's normal psychological development.[7] Parental separation during hospitalization has been associated with temporary and permanent detrimental effects on development.[8] Outpatient surgery may decrease the psychosocial impact of inpatient hospitalization and parental separation.[9] This decreased impact is particularly relevant to patients with musculoskeletal disorders, such as patients with connective tissue disorders or neuromuscular diseases, who may require multiple surgical procedures and anesthetics over the course of their development.[7]

In addition to the economic and psychological advantages, outpatient surgery has the potential to decrease other risks of hospitalization, such as nosocomial infection,[9] although this has not been demonstrated in clinical studies.

Surgeons may also benefit from increased outpatient procedures by creating less scheduling delays and allowing more autonomy.[10] These features are advantageous to hospitals as well in terms of bed and resource allocation.

CHALLENGES IN PEDIATRIC ORTHOPEDIC OUTPATIENT SURGERY

Although there are numerous advantages of outpatient orthopedic surgery in the pediatric population, several challenges exist to its universal implementation. These challenges may be medical, social, procedural, or environmental in nature.

Pediatric orthopedic patients represent a heterogeneous population with a variety of comorbidities. The anesthetic care of infants and young children is fundamentally different from those of adults and may require different specialized equipment and/or care providers.[8] Outpatient surgery centers that are not dedicated pediatric facilities may not be equipped with the appropriate resources to safely take care of pediatric patients. The exception to this could be older adolescent patients who may be physiologically similar to an adult.

A limiting factor in the practice of pediatric orthopedic outpatient surgery is achieving adequate pain control in the perioperative period. Although the increased rate of outpatient orthopedic surgery is in large part due to improved techniques for perioperative pain management, including regional anesthesia,[11] numerous studies and reviews have reported a significant percentage of patients with inadequate analgesia following several common ambulatory surgeries.[9,12–15] Pain remains difficult to assess objectively, especially in younger children; pediatric-specific pain teams, pediatric-specific pain assessment tools, and child-life specialists have been advocated as ways to help combat this challenge.[16] As opposed to inpatient hospitalization where pain can be regularly evaluated by pediatric-trained professionals and treated with a wide armamentarium of analgesics (oral and intravenous), pain evaluation and medication administration in outpatient surgery relies on a parent or caregiver who may have poor health literacy.[9] Automated mobile phone text messaging may offer providers opportunities to monitor postoperative pain and other symptoms as the volume of outpatient surgery increases.[17]

SUITABILITY OF OUTPATIENT SURGERY
Patient Factors

Preoperative screening is paramount to improving patient satisfaction and minimizing complications (including readmissions) with outpatient pediatric surgery.[18] A thorough history and physical is mandatory before any procedure. The American Society of Anesthesiologists' (ASA) physical status classification system (Table 1) may be used to classify patients according to the severity and stability of their medical comorbidities. ASA 1 and 2 patients are generally good candidates for outpatient surgery. Advanced preoperative evaluation by a member of the anesthesia team can help delineate a patient's medical suitability for outpatient surgery in equivocal case. ASA 3 patients with stable conditions may be candidates for outpatient procedures but are probably better cared for in centers with a capability for inpatient admission in the event of any perioperative complications. Overnight observation should be planned for ASA 4 patients.[19] Because of the complex medical comorbidities of many patients with orthopedic conditions, including pediatric patients, there will always be cases whereby care and

Table 1
American Society of Anesthesiologists'
physical status classification

ASA Class	Description
1	A healthy, normal patient
2	A patient with mild systemic disease
3	A patient with severe systemic disease that is not incapacitating
4	A patient with an incapacitating systemic disease that is a constant threat to life
5	A moribund patient with little chance of survival
E	A patient requiring an emergency operation

From American Society of Anesthesiologists: new classification of physical status. Anesthesiology 1963;24:111; with permission.

observation at an inpatient facility is required following anesthesia regardless of how benign or small the surgical procedure is. These patients frequently have neuromuscular disorders and/or cardiopulmonary comorbidities that require observation in an inpatient facility even in the setting of a relatively minor procedure.

Obstructive sleep apnea (OSA) affects approximately 1% to 6% of all children and up to 59% of children with obesity.[20] Patients with OSA are at an increased risk of respiratory events and apnea in the perioperative period given the influence of anesthetic agents, narcotics, and sedatives.[21] Although institutional polices vary, patients with OSA generally require additional monitoring in the postanesthesia care unit (PACU) and may require inpatient admission for monitoring and potential respiratory support.[20] All patients who are planned for outpatient pediatric surgery should be screened for snoring, mouth breathing, and sleep apnea–related symptoms suggestive of OSA.[20] Preoperative pulmonary consultation is recommended for patients with suspected OSA.

With respect to patient age, there is no consensus on a minimal age for safe outpatient surgery in infants.[22] Although minor procedures, such as Achilles tenotomy, can be safely performed in young infants on an outpatient basis, the authors recommend delaying larger elective procedures in patients until at least 6 months of age if possible.

Particular attention should be paid to patients' past surgical history to identify any prior difficulties with anesthesia, such as nausea,

vomiting, and poor pain control. This past experience may help guide the surgeon and anesthesiologist with respect to the perioperative anesthetic and analgesics plan as well as informing the surgeon about the suitability of parental care in the perioperative period.

Psychosocial Factors

In addition to the patients' overall medical status, the psychosocial background of patients and their living environment are critical to successful perioperative care. A preoperative social screen helps identify a patient's support network at home. This screen should identify the number and availability of caregivers at home, their comfort with providing basic care (eg, dressing changes, medication administration), availability of outpatient rehabilitation services, the physical environment of the household (eg, presence of stairs or physical barriers in the home), and travel needs. Patients who are traveling from significant distances may be poor candidates for outpatient surgery, particularly for cases that may end later in the day. The preoperative social screen is critical because the success of an operation is often contingent on safe and appropriate perioperative care.

Surgical Factors

The type, duration, and invasiveness of a surgical procedure play an important role in the safety of outpatient pediatric orthopedics. Of these factors, the invasiveness of the surgical procedure is likely the most important factor.[22] In general, bony procedures, such as osteotomies, carry the potential for more bleeding, swelling, and postoperative pain compared with purely soft tissue procedures. These considerations should be taken in the broader context of patients' underlying medical and psychosocial condition when determining suitability for an outpatient procedure.

Because of the elective nature of most outpatient surgeries, patients should be medically, socially, and psychologically optimized for planned procedures to increase outcomes and patient satisfaction.[18] A list of factors to consider regarding the suitability of outpatient pediatric orthopedic surgery is provided in Box 1.

ENVIRONMENT/SETTING FOR OUTPATIENT SURGERY

Ambulatory Surgery Centers

Pediatric outpatient surgery may be practiced in traditional inpatient venues or at dedicated outpatient facilities (eg, ambulatory surgery centers [ASCs]). Standalone ASCs tend to be

> **Box 1**
> **Factors to consider regarding the suitability of outpatient pediatric orthopedic surgery**
>
> - Patient medical status/ASA status/comorbidities (including obesity and/or OSA)
> - Patient social support and living situation
> - Anesthesia resources of care facility
> - Weight-bearing restrictions in the perioperative period
> - Potential complications of procedure
> - Whether there any advanced nursing needs in the perioperative setting
> - Whether the family/caregiver/patient understand activity restrictions/postoperative instructions

located in less urban environments compared with traditional children's hospitals, which may be attractive to patients and caregivers with respect to travel considerations (eg, transit time, parking, travel within the facility). Because of their smaller size and potential for increased specialization, the routine use of ASCs may lead to better allocation of medical personnel, equipment, and resources.[23]

A review of more than 1000 outpatient orthopedic procedures at the authors' institution found that outpatient surgery at a pediatric ASC rather than at a university children's hospital afforded a direct cost savings of 17% to 43% depending on the procedure performed. These cost savings were driven largely by reduced time expenditures in the operating room.[23] Improved cost accounting techniques (time-driven activity-based costing) that capture the true cost of labor and facility utilization have been developed and are uncovering other opportunities for cost savings in outpatient surgery.[24]

Utilization of ASCs in pediatric orthopedic care seems to be increasing rapidly. Bernstein and colleagues[25] queried the Centers for Disease Control and Prevention's national ambulatory surgery database and noted that the proportion of care being performed at freestanding ASCs increased by a factor of 7, from 3% to 21% between 1996 and 2006. This shift toward ASCs was observed in the context of increased use of outpatient surgery for pediatric fracture care, which increased threefold from 10% to 32% over the same period time.[25]

Although some patients with significant medical comorbidities (eg, ASA 3 or 4) may be poor

candidates for treatment at an ASC, the authors think that ASCs provide an opportunity for convenient outpatient orthopedic surgical care to a large proportion of patients in a fiscally responsible manner.

Avoiding the Operating Room Entirely

Occasionally orthopedic procedures may be treated outside of the operating room entirely. In doing so, they have the potential for significant time and cost savings.

Percutaneous Achilles tenotomy is performed for residual equinus contracture in approximately 80% of patients with clubfoot treated with the Ponseti method. Multiple investigators, including Ponseti, have described that performing this procedure in the outpatient/office setting with topical and/or local anesthesia is safe and effective.[26–29] Percutaneous Achilles tenotomy is not associated with a substantial rate of subsequent hospital admission or visits to the emergency department.

Another potential for avoiding the cost and time associated with procedures in the operating room is with nonoperative care of pediatric femur fractures. Numerous investigators have described spica cast application in the emergency department for select pediatric femur fractures with equivalent outcomes to patients managed in the operating room.[30–32] This technique may allow for earlier definitive treatment of children while avoiding the time and cost associated with operating room use. Mansour and colleagues[31] reviewed a cohort of patients with pediatric femur fractures who were treated with spica casting in the emergency department (n = 79) versus patients treated in the operating room (n = 21). Patients treated in the emergency department had significantly decreased time to cast placement (3.8 hours vs 11.5 hours, $P<.0001$), decreased length of stay (16.9 hours vs 30.5 hours, $P = .0002$), and decreased cost ($5150 vs $15,983, $P<.0001$) compared with patients treated in the emergency department.

PAIN MANAGEMENT STRATEGIES FOR OUTPATIENT SURGERY

As mentioned previously, pain is often a limiting factor in determining patients' suitability for outpatient pediatric orthopedic surgery. Recent advances in anesthetic techniques, particularly within regional anesthesia, have greatly improved analgesia in the perioperative period and may contribute to increasing the prevalence of pediatric ambulatory surgery.

Regional anesthesia refers to the targeted use of local anesthetics on neural structures to block afferent pain sensation. Regional anesthetics may be applied to a single nerve, a group of nerves, or via local infiltration. The overall experience for several ambulatory pediatric orthopedic procedures has been improved with regard to analgesia, safety, and perceived satisfaction with the use of regional anesthesia.[33]

Although regional anesthesia is often administered to awake adults with sedation, regional anesthesia in the pediatric population is often administered with patients under general anesthesia given concerns for patient anxiety and psychosocial well-being.[34] The safety of regional blocks administered to patients under general anesthesia has been demonstrated in a recent large series.[35] The use of ultrasound guidance allows for improved safety and precision when working around neural structures that are commonly in close proximity to other critical anatomic structures,[33] with complication rates of upper and lower extremity regional blocks in the pediatric population as low as 1% to 2%.[36]

Newer combinations of anesthetics with different pharmacokinetics allow for sustained duration of neural blockade, whereas nerve catheters allow for the continued injection of anesthetic over a period of time. The complication rate associated with pediatric nerve catheters is approximately 12%, with catheter dislodgement or block failure being the most frequent.[37] Despite this relatively high overall complication rate, the rate of serious complications is low (~0.04%), with no documented cases of permanent neurologic injury in pediatric patients.[33,37]

In addition to regional anesthetic techniques, there has been a recent movement from opioid-centric pathways to multimodal pain regimes. These regimens include multiple, nonopioid analgesics, such as acetaminophen or nonsteroidal antiinflammatories, along with regional anesthesia. Multimodal anesthesia has been associated with a diminished need for narcotics and a decrease in associated side effects.[9]

These multimodal strategies can lead to improved perioperative pain control and a decreased need for hospital admission following outpatient procedures. Hall-Burton and colleagues[34] found conversion from a primarily opioid-based pain management program to lower-extremity nerve blocks for postoperative pediatric ACL reconstruction pain was associated with a lower rate of unanticipated hospital admission (7% vs 18%, $P = .045$), less time in PACU phase II (145 minutes vs 192 minutes, $P = .013$), and a reduction in PACU opioid consumption (0.05 mg/kg vs 0.13 mg/kg, $P<.001$). This effect was independent of patient age, weight, or sex.

A common concern regarding regional anesthesia among orthopedic surgeons is the potential to increases the risk of acute compartment syndrome (ACS) in children by masking pain symptoms that would lead to expedient diagnosis and treatment. Current literature does not support this concern; however, this theoretic risk should be considered and discussed with patients and families.[38] If a surgeon has a concern for the potential for postoperative ACS, it should be discussed with the treating anesthesiologist, as this may influence the choice of regional anesthetic. The presence of breakthrough pain in the setting of a well-functioning block may be an early indicator of ACS and should evaluated seriously.[9]

READMISSION FOLLOWING OF OUTPATIENT SURGERY

Although outpatient surgery offers the potential for significant cost savings, these advantages are lost if patients require urgent or emergency care because of adverse events.[5] The incidence of unanticipated admission following all pediatric surgery is approximately 1%, with pediatric orthopedic cases demonstrating a significantly higher readmission rate (~2.5%). Approximately half of these readmissions are anesthesia related. Risk factors for readmission following outpatient surgery include patient age less than 2 years, duration of surgery great than 1 hour, surgery completion after 3 PM, presence of OSA, or patients who are ASA 3 class.[39] Surgeons should be aware of these risk factors and individual patient and surgical factors when considering perioperative outpatient management.

STRATEGIES FOR SUCCESSFUL OUTPATIENT PEDIATRIC ORTHOPEDICS

Strategies for successful outpatient pediatric orthopedics focus on optimizing and preparing patients and their families for the entire treatment course. A summary of these strategies is outlined in **Box 2**.

Preoperative education is associated with decreased anxiety and improved patient/family satisfaction.[18,40] Thorough preoperative education regarding the entire episode of care is important for all procedures, and it is particularly important in outpatient surgery where a parent or guardian will be acting as a medical caregiver

---

Box 2
Summary of strategies for effective outpatient pediatric orthopedic surgery

1. Proper patient selection
2. Thorough preoperative education and gait training
3. Multimodal analgesics (before, during, and after the procedure)
4. Close outpatient follow-up and communication
5. Ongoing surveillance and quality-improvement measures

---

during recovery. Parents/guardians should receive oral and written instructions regarding appropriate medications, including analgesics, regarding their dosing, schedule, and strategies for minimizing side effects. Providing postoperative prescriptions before surgery allows families to obtain pain medicines in advance, ensuring that no delays are encountered when traveling home.

Parents/guardians must understand symptoms and signs to look out for in the perioperative setting that may require medical care or intervention. Parents/guardians and patients should understand any activity or weight-bearing restrictions, and mobility should be rehearsed before the day of surgery. A one-time appointment with a physical and/or occupational therapist may be instrumental in ensuring safe mobility at home following surgery.

Parents/guardians should be provided with information regarding how to contact a member of the medical team should any questions or concerns arise. A routine follow-up call the day after surgery from a member of the surgical team provides an opportunity to check in and can improve patient satisfaction. Data regarding postoperative patient pain control, satisfaction, and safety should be shared in a multidisciplinary fashion in order to improve practice patterns.

Before discharge from the PACU, patients should have acceptable pain control, be able to tolerate oral liquids and nourishment, and have safe and acceptable mobility.[18]

If an ambulatory surgery center is used, a contingency plan must be available should situations arise whereby patients cannot be safely discharged home. Often this is accomplished in the form of a relationship with a neighboring hospital where the attending surgeon has admitting privileges should the need arise.[18]

FUTURE DIRECTIONS

Outpatient pediatric surgery is still in infant stages, and routine use is still exploratory at this time. Continuous research in quality, value, and patient safety is needed to ensure that this practice continues to develop in as safe and efficient a manner as possible.[18]

SUMMARY

For many pediatric orthopedic procedures, outpatient surgery may offer a realistic, safe, and efficient alternative to inpatient perioperative management. Evidence-based multidisciplinary efforts can lead to decreased pain, decreased morbidity, fewer unplanned readmissions, and increased patient satisfaction following outpatient pediatric orthopedic surgery while decreasing costs to the medical system as a whole. However, it is important to remember that outpatient surgery is not a universal *best choice* solution for pediatric orthopedic surgery. The decision for inpatient versus outpatient perioperative management should be tailored to each patient and family in a patient-focused model.

REFERENCES

1. Crawford DC, Li CS, Sprague S, et al. Clinical and cost implications of inpatient versus outpatient orthopedic surgeries: a systematic review of the published literature. Orthop Rev (Pavia) 2015;7(4):6177.
2. Brolin TJ, Mulligan RP, Azar FM, et al. Neer Award 2016: outpatient total shoulder arthroplasty in an ambulatory surgery center is a safe alternative to inpatient total shoulder arthroplasty in a hospital: a matched cohort study. J Shoulder Elbow Surg 2017;26(2):204–8.
3. Rabbitts JA, Groenewald CB, Moriarty JP, et al. Epidemiology of ambulatory anesthesia for children in the United States: 2006 and 1996. Anesth Analg 2010;111(4):1011–5.
4. August DA, Everett LL. Pediatric ambulatory anesthesia. Anesthesiol Clin 2014;32(2):411–29.
5. Martin-Ferrero MA, Faour-Martin O, Simon-Perez C, et al. Ambulatory surgery in orthopedics: experience of over 10,000 patients. J Orthop Sci 2014;19(2):332–8.
6. Porter ME. What is value in health care? N Engl J Med 2010;363(26):2477–81.
7. Zuckerberg AL, Yaster M. Anesthesia for Pediatric Orthopedic Surgery. In: Davis PJ, Cladis FP, editors. Smith's Anesthesia for Infants and Children. 9th edition. Philadelphia: Elsevier; 2017. p. 865–91.

8. Davis PJ, Motoyama EK, Cladis FP. Special Characteristics of Pediatric Anesthesia. In: Davis PJ, Cladis FP, editors. Smith's Anesthesia for Infants and Children. 9th edition. Philadelphia: Elsevier; 2017. p. 2–9.

9. Stein AL, Baumgard D, Del Rio I, et al. Updates in pediatric regional anesthesia and its role in the treatment of acute pain in the ambulatory setting. Curr Pain Headache Rep 2017;21(2):11.

10. Kao JT, Giangarra CE, Singer G, et al. A comparison of outpatient and inpatient anterior cruciate ligament reconstruction surgery. Arthroscopy 1995; 11(2):151–6.

11. Kuo C, Edwards A, Mazumdar M, et al. Regional anesthesia for children undergoing orthopedic ambulatory surgeries in the United States, 1996-2006. HSS J 2012;8(2):133–6.

12. Mather L, Mackie J. The incidence of postoperative pain in children. Pain 1983;15(3):271–82.

13. Wolf AR. Tears at bedtime: a pitfall of extending paediatric day-case surgery without extending analgesia. Br J Anaesth 1999;82(3):319–20.

14. Dorkham MC, Chalkiadis GA, von Ungern Sternberg BS, et al. Effective postoperative pain management in children after ambulatory surgery, with a focus on tonsillectomy: barriers and possible solutions. Paediatr Anaesth 2014;24(3):239–48.

15. Shum S, Lim J, Page T, et al. An audit of pain management following pediatric day surgery at British Columbia Children's Hospital. Pain Res Manag 2012;17(5):328–34.

16. Nowicki PD, Vanderhave KL, Gibbons K, et al. Perioperative pain control in pediatric patients undergoing orthopaedic surgery. J Am Acad Orthop Surg 2012;20(12):755–65.

17. Anthony CA, Peterson AR. Utilization of a text-messaging robot to assess intraday variation in concussion symptom severity scores. Clin J Sport Med 2015;25(2):149–52.

18. Argenson JN, Husted H, Lombardi A Jr, et al. Global forum: an international perspective on outpatient surgical procedures for adult hip and knee reconstruction. J Bone Joint Surg Am 2016;98(13):e55.

19. Emhardt JD, Saysana C, Sirichotvithyakorn P. Anesthetic considerations for pediatric outpatient surgery. Semin Pediatr Surg 2004;13(3):210–21.

20. Schwengel DA, Dalesio NM, Stierer TL. Pediatric obstructive sleep apnea. Anesthesiol Clin 2014; 32(1):237–61.

21. Wolfe RM, Pomerantz J, Miller DE, et al. Obstructive sleep apnea: preoperative screening and postoperative care. J Am Board Fam Med 2016;29(2):263–75.

22. Johr M, Berger TM. Anaesthesia for the paediatric outpatient. Curr Opin Anaesthesiol 2015;28(6):623–30.

23. Fabricant PD, Seeley MA, Rozell JC, et al. Cost savings from utilization of an ambulatory surgery center for orthopaedic day surgery. J Am Acad Orthop Surg 2016;24(12):865–71.

24. Kaplan RS, Witkowski M, Abbott M, et al. Using time-driven activity-based costing to identify value improvement opportunities in healthcare. J Healthc Manag 2014;59(6):399–412.

25. Bernstein DT, Chen C, Zhang W, et al. National trends in operative treatment of pediatric fractures in the ambulatory setting. Orthopedics 2015;38(10):e869–73.

26. Lebel E, Karasik M, Bernstein-Weyel M, et al. Achilles tenotomy as an office procedure: safety and efficacy as part of the Ponseti serial casting protocol for clubfoot. J Pediatr Orthop 2012;32(4):412–5.

27. Willis RB, Al-Hunaishel M, Guerra L, et al. What proportion of patients need extensive surgery after failure of the Ponseti technique for clubfoot? Clin Orthop Relat Res 2009;467(5):1294–7.

28. Ponseti I. Congenital clubfoot, fundamentals of treatment. Great Britain (United Kingdom): Oxford University Press; 1996.

29. Alam MT, Akber EB, Alam QS, et al. Outcome of percutaneous tenotomy in the management of congenital talipes equinovarus by Ponseti method. Mymensingh Med J 2015;24(3):467–70.

30. Cassinelli EH, Young B, Vogt M, et al. Spica cast application in the emergency room for select pediatric femur fractures. J Orthop Trauma 2005;19(10):709–16.

31. Mansour AA 3rd, Wilmoth JC, Mansour AS, et al. Immediate spica casting of pediatric femoral fractures in the operating room versus the emergency department: comparison of reduction, complications, and hospital charges. J Pediatr Orthop 2010;30(8):813–7.

32. Infante AF Jr, Albert MC, Jennings WB, et al. Immediate hip spica casting for femur fractures in pediatric patients. A review of 175 patients. Clin Orthop Relat Res 2000;(376):106–12.

33. Deer JD, Sawardekar A, Suresh S. Day surgery regional anesthesia in children: safety and improving outcomes, do they make a difference? Curr Opin Anaesthesiol 2016;29(6):691–5.

34. Hall-Burton DM, Hudson ME, Grudziak JS, et al. Regional anesthesia is cost-effective in preventing unanticipated hospital admission in pediatric patients having anterior cruciate ligament reconstruction. Reg Anesth Pain Med 2016;41(4):527–31.

35. Taenzer AH, Walker BJ, Bosenberg AT, et al. Asleep versus awake: does it matter?: pediatric regional block complications by patient state: a report from the Pediatric Regional Anesthesia Network. Reg Anesth Pain Med 2014;39(4):279–83.

36. Polaner DM, Taenzer AH, Walker BJ, et al. Pediatric Regional Anesthesia Network (PRAN): a multi-institutional study of the use and incidence of

complications of pediatric regional anesthesia. Anesth Analg 2012;115(6):1353–64.

37. Walker BJ, Long JB, De Oliveira GS, et al. Peripheral nerve catheters in children: an analysis of safety and practice patterns from the pediatric regional anesthesia network (PRAN). Br J Anaesth 2015; 115(3):457–62.

38. Ivani G, Suresh S, Ecoffey C, et al. The European Society of Regional Anaesthesia and Pain Therapy and the American Society of Regional Anesthesia and Pain Medicine Joint Committee Practice Advisory on Controversial Topics in Pediatric Regional Anesthesia. Reg Anesth Pain Med 2015; 40(5):526–32.

39. Whippey A, Kostandoff G, Ma HK, et al. Predictors of unanticipated admission following ambulatory surgery in the pediatric population: a retrospective case-control study. Paediatr Anaesth 2016;26(8): 831–7.

40. Yoon RS, Nellans KW, Geller JA, et al. Patient education before hip or knee arthroplasty lowers length of stay. J Arthroplasty 2010;25(4):547–51.

Hand and Wrist

Use of Wide-awake Local Anesthesia No Tourniquet in Hand and Wrist Surgery

Murphy M. Steiner, MD[a],*, James H. Calandruccio, MD[b]

KEYWORDS

- Local anesthesia • Hand surgery • Epinephrine • Outcomes • Complications

KEY POINTS

- Local anesthesia is used for most surgical procedures in the hand and wrist, but generally requires the use of a tourniquet to obtain a "bloodless field."
- The addition of epinephrine in the WALANT (wide-awake local anesthesia no tourniquet) technique achieves acceptable vision without the use of a tourniquet.
- Epinephrine has been proven safe for use in hand and digits.
- Patient satisfaction is high, and savings in time and costs are substantial.

Local and regional anesthesia techniques have been used for hand surgeries for many years, with general anesthesia typically reserved for extensive and prolonged hand operations, especially in young children. There are well-known risks associated with general and regional anesthesia, such as allergic reactions and systemic toxic effects, and some patients have comorbidities that are contraindications to general or regional anesthesia.[1] Because of these issues, local infiltration of anesthetic agents is commonly used for many surgical procedures of the hand and wrist. A newer technique currently being used by more and more hand surgeons is THE "wide-awake local anesthesia no tourniquet" (WALANT).[2,3]

THE EPINEPHRINE MYTH

WALANT uses a combination of a local anesthetic such as lidocaine or bupivacaine and epinephrine to induce anesthesia and hemostasis in the area of the surgical procedure. For many years, epinephrine was thought to cause devastating complications, including necrosis and gangrene, when used for hand or foot surgery. More recently, however, several studies and reviews of older literature have shown that this is not the case.[4] A multicenter prospective study of 3110 consecutive patients who had epinephrine injections into the hands or fingers found that none produced any skin necrosis or digital tissue loss of any kind.[5] Three literature reviews[6–8] found no valid evidence to support the concept that lidocaine with epinephrine is not safe for injection into the fingers; the authors found no reports of digital infarction. Several early series also reported the safe use of epinephrine injections in the hand and wrist. Johnson[9] reported no ill effects with the injection of epinephrine in 421 hands and fingers; Denkler[10] described fasciectomies in 60 consecutive digits using lidocaine with epinephrine and no tourniquet with no resulting ischemia, and Wilhelmi and colleagues[11] reported no complications in 30 procedures done with lidocaine and epinephrine. Further supporting the safety of epinephrine injection is the study by

Disclosure Statement: Neither Dr J.H. Calandruccio nor Dr M.M. Steiner has anything to disclose.
[a] Department of Hand Surgery, Bienville Orthopaedic Specialists, 6300 East Lake Boulevard, Gautier, MS 39565, USA; [b] Department of Orthopaedic Surgery and Biomedical Engineering, University of Tennessee-Campbell Clinic, 1211 Union Avenue, Suite 510, Memphis, TN 38104, USA
* Corresponding author.
E-mail address: murphysteiner@gmail.com

Fitzcharles-Bowe and colleagues,[7] in which they described 59 instances of high-dose (1:1000) digital epinephrine injection. This concentration is 100 times larger than that used for WALANT, and none of the digits had necrosis or tissue loss.

ADVANTAGES OF WIDE-AWAKE LOCAL ANESTHESIA NO TOURNIQUET FOR PATIENTS

WALANT has several advantages for use in the hand and fingers (Box 1). The primary advantage is the avoidance of the use of a tourniquet, which reduces patient discomfort and avoids the risk of temporary or permanent nerve and skin injury from the tourniquet. No overnight fasting, preoperative testing, or anesthesia consult is required; no intravenous catheter is needed, and minimal draping and instrumentation are required. Because the awake patient can actively move his or her hand or wrist, the function and stability of repairs and reconstructions can be evaluated intraoperatively and any necessary adjustments can be made. Recovery time is minimized, and, because side effects that are common with anesthesia (eg, nausea, grogginess) are avoided, most procedures done with WALANT can be done as outpatient procedures. Patient satisfaction is high with this anesthesia method.[12] Rhee and colleagues[13] reported that 62 (94%) of 66 patients surveyed

would choose it for any future hand surgeries, and Davison and colleagues[14] reported similar results in 100 patients who had carpal tunnel release (93% would prefer WALANT over intravenous or general anesthesia). In a comparison of sedated and wide-awake patients who had carpal tunnel releases, most were satisfied with whichever method of anesthesia they received, but sedated patients were in the hospital longer, required more preoperative testing, and reported more preoperative anxiety.[14] Postoperative narcotics were used by 5% of wide-awake patients and by 67% of sedated patients. A recent study by Hustedt and colleagues[15] compared 4614 patients who had hand surgery with local/regional anesthesia without sedation, 3527 who had local/regional anesthesia with sedation, and 18,900 who had general anesthesia. Overall, both local and regional anesthesia with and without sedation had fewer postoperative complications than general anesthesia. In patients older than 65 years, there was the added benefit of avoiding all forms of sedation and decreasing the odds of postoperative complications. Data from this large nationwide study suggest that using local/regional anesthesia without sedation instead of general anesthesia reduces the odds of sustaining a postoperative complication after hand surgery by 1.5 times in patients of all ages and by 3.5 times in patients older than 65 years.

ADMINISTRATION OF WIDE-AWAKE LOCAL ANESTHESIA NO TOURNIQUET

Depending on the site at which dissection will occur, approximately 2 mL of 1% lidocaine with epinephrine 1:100,000 is injected into the palmar and dorsal subcutaneous tissues (Fig. 1). If hemostasis is not required and only a sensory block is needed, a single subcutaneous injection in the midline of the proximal phalanx with lidocaine and epinephrine (SIMPLE technique) is sufficient (see Fig. 1A). For procedures in the distal phalanx, Lalonde and Wong[16] recommend no more than 1 mL (Box 2).

Although some literature supports the safe use of 35 mg/kg of lidocaine with epinephrine,[17] the generally accepted maximal dose is 7 mg/kg,[16] meaning that an approximately 150-pound patient can safely receive 50 mL, which is well over the amount recommended for common hand and wrist procedures (Table 1).

Bupivacaine is preferred over lidocaine by some because of its longer duration of action, although the pain block provided by

---

Box 1
Advantages of wide-awake local anesthesia no tourniquet for patients

- No sedation or general anesthesia
  - No side effects, such as nausea, vomiting, grogginess
- No anesthesiologist
  - Lower cost, less time
- No overnight fasting
  - Especially important for diabetic patients
- No presurgery testing
  - Saves times and money
- No intravenous line
- No tourniquet
  - Less pain
- Faster recovery
  - Outpatient procedure in clinic or surgery center
- Fewer complications

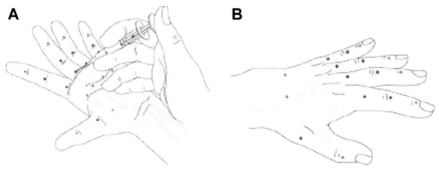

Fig. 1. Sites of injection of local anesthesia in finger and hand surgery. (*A*) Volar injections. When only a sensory block of the finger is required (SIMPLE technique), 2 mL is injected into the areas designated by the blue dots. To obtain hemostasis and local anesthesia for palmar finger surgery, 1% lidocaine with epinephrine 1:100,000 is injected into the midline subcutaneous fat between the digital nerve in each area designated by a dot. (*B*) Dorsal injections. For hemostasis and local anesthesia, injection is made into the midline subcutaneous fat in each area designated by a dot. In both volar and dorsal injections, 2 mL is injected at the site of blue and red dots, 1 mL at the site of the green dots, and 5 mL at the site of the orange dots. (*From* Lalonde D, Martin A. Epinephrine in local anesthesia in finger and hand surgery: the case for wide-awake anesthesia. J Am Acad Orthop Surg 2013;21(8):445; with permission.)

Box 2
Tips for administering wide-awake local anesthesia no tourniquet

- Pain during administration can be reduced by several methods

  - Buffering the solution: a solution of lidocaine 1% with 1:100,000 epinephrine has a pH 4.2, which likely contributes to the pain with injection.[22,23] A 1:20 ratio of 8.4% sodium bicarbonate to lidocaine 1% with 1:100,000 epinephrine has a more physiologic pH 7.4. A *Cochrane Review*[24] concluded that patients much preferred buffered lidocaine to unbuffered lidocaine; the difference was even more pronounced when the solution contained epinephrine.

  - Warming the solution.[25–27]

  - Using a smaller needle (27- or 30-gauge or smaller).[28]

  - Choosing the correct angle for needle insertion: A randomized, controlled crossover trial of 65 patients showed that injections with needles oriented at 90° were significantly less painful than those with needles oriented at 45°.[29]

  - Injecting the solution under the dermis: In their double-blind, prospective trial, Arndt and colleagues[30] found that subdermal injections produced less pain than intradermal injections. Strazar and colleagues[23] suggested that this occurred because the space-occupying effect of the solution stretches the tissue, producing more pain in the densely innervated dermal tissue.

bupivacaine lasts about half as long (15 hours) as the return to normal sensation (30 hours), and adding epinephrine prolongs the duration of pain relief for only an additional 1.5 hours.[18] Patients need to be informed that pain sensation will return much sooner than numbness will resolve. With lidocaine, pain and sensation return simultaneously. Most hand operations can be done in the anesthesia time provided by lidocaine with epinephrine (5 hours in the wrist, 10 hours in the finger). Bupivacaine may be preferable for operations that last more than 2.5 to 3 hours and after which pain may be severe.

Although it was long thought that the time to maximal vasoconstriction after injection of lidocaine and epinephrine was 7 minutes, it has now been shown that this does not occur until at least 25 minutes after injection.[19] Bashir and colleagues[20] randomized 75 patients to 10-, 15-, or 25-minute intervals between infiltration and incision and found that an interval of 25 minutes provided vastly superior operative field visibility, whereas 10-minute delay had the poorest results. McKee and colleagues[19,21] recommend waiting approximately 30 minutes before incision for maximal hemostasis.

SPECIFIC PROCEDURES SUITABLE FOR WIDE-AWAKE LOCAL ANESTHESIA NO TOURNIQUET

Flexor Tendon Repair

The use of WALANT for flexor tendon repair allows voluntary active motion by the patient, which may exhibit gapping of the repair site

Table 1
Typical volumes used for common operations (1% lidocaine with 1:100,000 epinephrine and 8.4% bicarbonate, mixed 10 mL:1 mL)

Operation	Volume	Location
Carpal tunnel	20 mL	10 mL between ulnar and median nerves (5 mm proximal to wrist crease and 5 mm ulnar to median nerve); another 10 mL under incision
Trigger finger	4 mL	Subcutaneously beneath the center of the incision
Finger sensory block (SIMPLE)	2 mL	Volar middle of proximal phalanx just past palmar-finger crease
Finger soft tissue lesions or other surgery in which finger-base tourniquet is not desirable and finger epinephrine is used for hemostasis	5 mL volar distributed among 3 phalanges, 4 mL dorsal split between 2 phalanges	2 mL volar and 2 mL dorsal subcutaneous midline fat, in both proximal and middle phalanges; only 1 mL in the distal phalanx, midline volar, just past the DIP crease
PIP arthrodesis	8 mL total, 4 mL volar (2 in each phalanx) and 4 mL dorsal (2 in each phalanx)	2 mL midvolar and another 2 mL middorsal of both proximal and middle phalanges
Thumb MCP arthrodesis and collateral ligament tears of the MCP joint	15 mL	2 mL on each of volar and dorsal aspects of the proximal phalanx and the rest all around the metacarpal head
Dupuytren contracture or zone II flexor tendon repair	15 mL/ray	10 mL (or more) in the palm, then 2 mL in the proximal and middle phalanges and 1 mL in the distal phalanx (if required)
Trapeziectomy or Bennet fracture	40 mL	Radial side of the hand under the skin and all around the joint, including the median nerve. If LRTI is performed, the concentration is decreased to 0.5% lidocaine and 1:200,000 epinephrine and also is injected all around where FCR or APL will be dissected
Metacarpal fractures	40 mL	All around the metacarpal where dissection or K-wire insertion will occur

Abbreviations: APL, abductor pollicis longus; DIP, distal interphalangeal joint; FCR, flexor carpi radialis; LRTI, ligament reconstruction and tendon interposition; MCP, metacarpophalangeal joint; PIP, proximal interphalangeal joint; SIMPLE, single subcutaneous injection in the middle of the proximal phalanx with lidocaine and epinephrine.
Modified from Lalonde DH, Wong A. Dosage of local anesthesia in wide awake hand surgery. J Hand Surg Am 2013;38(10):2027; with permission.

and allow immediate intraoperative augmentation or revision.[31–33] It also allows the surgeon to make intraoperative decisions on pulley management by observing smooth gliding of pulleys that might have otherwise been sacrificed. Patient education and rehabilitation can begin immediately after surgery because active total motion is observed in the operating room (OR).

Tendon Transfer
For tendon transfer to be successful, the transferred tendon must be appropriately tensioned. WALANT allows observation of the tendon transfer in action before definitive fixation.[34]

Releases
Soft tissue releases are used for a variety of hand conditions, such as trigger finger and De Quervain tenosynovitis, and complete release of the appropriate soft tissues can be confirmed intraoperatively with active motion.

Hagert and Lalonde[35] described the use of WALANT for arthroscopic and open triangular fibrocartilage repair in 9 patients, and Sørensen and colleagues[36] reported endoscopic carpal tunnel release in 38 patients with the use of local anesthesia. Rhee and colleagues[13] also reported successful use of WALANT for pin fixation of phalangeal fractures, hardware/foreign body removal, and nail horn excision/ablation.

COST SAVINGS AND EFFICIENCY

Elimination of the need for a tourniquet with WALANT also eliminates the need for sedation, monitoring, and a full OR. Patients do not require preoperative testing, including blood work, chest radiographs, electrocardiogram, and medical clearance. The procedure can be done in a procedure room with field sterility. The patient does not need to change clothes, and the surgeon does not need to wear a gown, but should wear a mask and sterile gloves. Only a simple tray of sterile surgical instruments is necessary. Recovery room time is significantly reduced.

With increased pressure on hospitals to decrease costs and increase efficiency, several studies have examined the role of reducing turnover time to increase throughput in the OR. Caggiano and colleagues[37] evaluated nonsurgical time, defined as the time elapsed from surgery end time for one patient until the surgery start time for the next patient, according to type of anesthesia used. The choice of anesthesia had a significant effect on room turnover time, in-room presurgical time, in-room postsurgical time, and total nonsurgical time. Local-only anesthesia reduced total nonsurgical time by 40% compared with general anesthesia and by 24% compared with monitored (local or general) anesthesia.

In a detailed analysis of direct costs for open carpal tunnel release, Leblanc and colleagues[38] determined that carpal tunnel release in an ambulatory setting cost one-fourth of the same procedure in the hospital OR. In addition, during a 3-hour surgical block time, 9 procedures were done in the ambulatory setting compared with 4 in the hospital OR. Nelson and colleagues[39] compared the cost of fasciectomy for Dupuytren contracture in an ambulatory setting to that in the hospital OR and concluded that costs in the OR were 13 times more than in the ambulatory setting. Chatterjee and colleagues[40] reported that the cost of an open carpal tunnel release in the OR ($2273) was nearly 4 times more expensive than in the clinic ($985) in a US tertiary health care center. Bismil and colleagues[41] determined that a "one-stop wide-awake hand surgery service" saved the British National Health Service more than $2 million in the last 10 years. Most recently, Rhee and colleagues,[13] in a prospective cohort study, analyzed the first 100 clinic-based, WALANT procedures done at a military medical center. They found a cost savings of 85% for carpal tunnel release and 70% for A1 pulley release compared with the same procedures done in the hospital OR, for a cost savings of nearly $400,000 over 21 months.

SUMMARY

WALANT appears to be a safe and effective anesthesia technique for many hand and wrist surgeries. Patient satisfaction is high because of the avoidance of preoperative testing and hospital admission. Postoperative recovery is rapid, and procedures can be done in outpatient settings, resulting in substantial savings in time and money.

REFERENCES

1. Auroy Y, Benhamou D, Bargues L, et al. Major complications of regional anesthesia in France. Anesthesiology 2002;97:1274–80.
2. Lalonde D, Eaton C, Amadio PC, et al. Wide-awake hand and wrist surgery: a new horizon in outpatient surgery. Instr Course Lect 2015;64:249–59.
3. Lalonde D, Martin A. Epinephrine in local anesthesia in finger and hand surgery: the case for wide-awake anesthesia. J Am Acad Orthop Surg 2013;21:443–7.
4. Cantlon MB, Yang SS. Wide awake hand surgery. Bull Hosp Jt Dis 2017;75:47–51.
5. Lalonde D, Bell M, Benoit P, et al. A multicenter prospective study of 3,110 consecutive cases of elective epinephrine use in the fingers and hand: the Dalhousie Project clinical phase. J Hand Surg 2005;30A:1061–7.
6. Denkler K. A comprehensive review of epinephrine in the finger: to do or not to do. Plast Reconstr Surg 2001;108:114–24.
7. Fitzcharles-Bowe C, Denkler K, Lalonde D. Finger injection with high-dose (1:1,000) epinephrine: does it cause finger necrosis and should it be treated? Hand (N Y) 2007;2:5–11.
8. Thomson CJ, Lalonde DH, Denkler FA, et al. A critical look at the evidence for and against elective epinephrine use in the finger. Plast Reconstr Surg 2007;119:260–6.
9. Johnson HA. Infiltration with epinephrine and local anesthetic mixture in the hand. JAMA 1967;200:990–1.
10. Denkler K. Dupuytren's fasciectomies in 60 consecutive digits using lidocaine with epinephrine and no tourniquet. Plast Reconstr Surg 2005;115:801–10.
11. Wilhelmi BJ, Blackwell SJ, Miller JS, et al. Do not use epinephrine in digital blocks: myth or truth? Plast Reconstr Surg 2001;107:393–7.
12. Lalonde D, Martin A. Tumescent local anesthesia for hand surgery: improved results, cost effectiveness,

and wide-awake patient satisfaction. Arch Plast Surg 2014;41:312–6.

13. Rhee PC, Fischer MM, Rhee LS, et al. Cost savings and patient experiences of a clinic-based, wide-awake hand surgery program at a military medical center: a critical analysis of the first 100 procedures. J Hand Surg Am 2017;42:e139–47.

14. Davison PG, Cobb T, Lalonde DH. The patient's perspective on carpal tunnel surgery related to the type of anesthesia: a prospective cohort study. Hand (N Y) 2013;8:47–53.

15. Hustedt JW, Chung A, Bohl DD, et al. Comparison of postoperative complications associated with anesthetic choice for surgery of the hand. J Hand Surg Am 2017;42:1–8.

16. Lalonde DH, Wong A. Dosage of local anesthesia in wide awake hand surgery. J Hand Surg 2013; 38A:2025–8.

17. Klein JA. Tumescent technique for regional anesthesia permits lidocaine doses of 35 mg/kg for liposuction. J Dermatol Surg Oncol 1990;16:248–63.

18. Calder K, Chung B, O'Brien C, et al. Bupivacaine digital blocks: how long is the pain relief and temperature elevation? Plast Reconstr Surg 2013;131: 1098–104.

19. McKee DE, Lalonde DH, Thoma A, et al. Optimal time delay between epinephrine injection and incision to minimize bleeding. Plast Reconstr Surg 2013;131:811–4.

20. Bashir MM, Oayyum R, Saleem MH, et al. Effect of time interval between tumescent local anesthesia infiltration and start of surgery on operative field visibility in hand surgery without tourniquet. J Hand Surg Am 2015;40:1606–9.

21. McKee DE, Lalonde DH, Thoma A, et al. Achieving the optimal epinephrine effect in wide awake hand surgery using local anesthesia without a tourniquet. Hand (N Y) 2005;10:613–5.

22. Lee HJ, Cho YJ, Gong HS, et al. The effect of buffered lidocaine in local anesthesia: a prospective, randomized double-blind study. J Hand Surg Am 2013;38:971–5.

23. Strazar AR, Leynes PG, Lalonde DH. Minimizing the pain of local anesthesia injection. Plast Reconstr Surg 2013;132:675–84.

24. Cepeda MS, Tzortzopoulou A, Thackeery M, et al. Adjusting the pH of lidocaine for reducing pain on injection. Cochrane Database Syst Rev 2010;(12):CD006581.

25. Hogan ME, vanderVaart S, Perampaladas K, et al. Systematic review and meta-analysis of the effect of warming local anesthetics on injection pain. Ann Emerg Med 2011;58:86–98.

26. Mader TJ, Playe SJ, Garb JL. Reducing the pain of local anesthetic infiltration: warming and buffering have a synergistic effect. Ann Emerg Med 1994; 23:550–4.

27. Yang CH, Hsu HC, Shen SC, et al. Warm and neutral tumescent anesthetic solutions are essential factors for a less painful injection. Dermatol Surg 2006;32:1119–22.

28. Arendt-Nielsen L, Egekvist H, Bjerring P. Pain following controlled cutaneous insertion of needles with different diameters. Somatosens Mot Res 2006;23:37–43.

29. Martires KJ, Malbasa CL, Bordeaux JS. A randomized controlled crossover trial: lidocaine injected at a 90-degree angle causes less pain than lidocaine injected at a 45-degree angle. J Am Acad Dermatol 2011;65:1231–3.

30. Arndt KA, Burton C, Noe JM. Minimizing the pain of local anesthesia. Plast Reconstr Surg 1983;73: 676–9.

31. Al Youha S, Lalonde DH. Update/review: changing of use of local anesthesia in the hand. Plast Reconstr Surg Glob Open 2014;2:e150.

32. Lalonde DH, Martin AL. Wide-awake flexor tendon repair and early tendon mobilization in zones 1 and 2. Hand Clin 2013;29:207–13.

33. Tang JB. Wide-awake primary flexor tendon repair, tenolysis, and tendon transfer. Clin Orthop Surg 2015;7:275–81.

34. Lalonde DH. Wide-awake extensor indicis proprius to extensor pollicis longus tendon transfer. J Hand Surg Am 2014;39:2297–9.

35. Hagert E, Lalonde DH. Wide-awake wrist arthroscopy and open TFCC repair. J Wrist Surg 2012;1: 55–60.

36. Sørensen AM, Dalsgaard J, Hansen TB. Local anaesthesia versus intravenous regional anesthesis in endoscopic carpal tunnel release:a randomized controlled trial. J Hand Surg Eur Vol 2013;38: 481–4.

37. Caggiano NM, Avery DM 3rd, Matullo KS. The effect of anesthesia type on nonsurgical operating room time. J Hand Surg Am 2015;40:1202–9.

38. Leblanc MR, Lalonde J, Lalonde DH. A detailed cost and efficiency analysis of performing carpal tunnel surgery in the main operating room versus the ambulatory setting in Canada. Hand (N Y) 2007;2(4):173–8.

39. Nelson R, Higgins A, Conrad J, et al. The wide-awake approach to Dupuytren's disease: fasciectomy under local anesthetic with epinephrine. Hand (N Y) 2010;5:117–24.

40. Chatterjee A, McCarthy JE, Montagne SA, et al. A cost, profit, and efficiency analysis of performing carpal tunnel surgery in the operating room versus the clinic setting in the United States. Ann Plast Surg 2011;66:245–8.

41. Bismil MSK, Bismil OMK, Harding D, et al. Transition to total one-stop wide-awake hand surgery service-audit: a retrospective review. JRSM Short Rep 2013;3:23.

Hand Surgery in the Ambulatory Surgery Center

Norfleet B. Thompson, MD,
James H. Calandruccio, MD*

KEYWORDS

- Hand surgery • Ambulatory surgery center • Costs • Complications

---

KEY POINTS

- A large percentage of hand surgery is done in ambulatory surgery centers (ASCs).
- Use of an ASC is more cost-effective and efficient than surgery in an inpatient facility.
- The complication rates are lower after surgery in an ASC than after surgery in an inpatient facility.
- Adequate postoperative pain control is essential to patient satisfaction.

Outpatient surgery, especially in free-standing ambulatory surgery centers (ASCs), provides a safe, cost-effective option for a variety of surgical procedures and has become the preferred choice over inpatient and hospital-based outpatient surgery for most hand and wrist procedures. According to a 2010 report from the US Centers for Disease Control and Prevention,[1] an estimated 48.3 million surgical procedures were done in hospital outpatient facilities or ASCs; 15% of these (7.1 million) were operations on the musculoskeletal system. Based on Medicare claims, approximately 7% of all procedures done at ASCs were orthopedic procedures.[2] A 2015 survey of American Society for Surgery of the Hand members found that 65% of hand surgeons reported doing most of their surgery at an ASC.[3] In their analysis of carpal tunnel release (CTR) in ASCs, Fajardo and colleagues[4] outlined the steady increase in the use of ASCs for CTR: in 1996, 16% of all ambulatory CTRs were done in freestanding ASCs; 10 years later the percentage was 49%. Patel and colleagues,[5] using data from the National Survey of Ambulatory Surgery, found a dramatic increase in the volume of ambulatory surgery (505%) for upper extremity fractures from 1996 to 2006. In most free-standing ASCs, hand and upper extremity surgeries are the primary procedures.[6] CTR, trigger finger release, tenosynovectomy (de Quervain), and fasciectomy (Dupuytren) are among the hand and wrist procedures frequently done in an ASC. Other, less frequently done procedures include flexor tendon repair, tendon transfers, fracture fixation, and interposition arthroplasty.

COSTS OF HAND SURGERY IN AN AMBULATORY SURGERY CENTER COMPARED WITH A HOSPITAL

One of the drivers of the boom in ASC surgery has been cost. The US Medicare fee schedule indicates that hospital outpatient surgical facilities are paid 81% more than ASCs for the same service.[6] Use of an ASC or office procedure room has been shown to decrease costs of hand surgery. CTR in an ambulatory setting has been determined to cost 25% to 30% less than the same procedure in the hospital operating room (OR),[7-9] in addition to allowing more than twice the number of procedures during a 3-hour

---

Department of Orthopaedic Surgery and Biomedical Engineering, University of Tennessee-Campbell Clinic, 1211 Union Avenue, Suite 510, Memphis, TN 38104, USA
* Corresponding author.
E-mail address: jcalandruccio@campbellclinic.com

Orthop Clin N Am 49 (2018) 69–72
http://dx.doi.org/10.1016/j.ocl.2017.08.009
0030-5898/18/© 2017 Elsevier Inc. All rights reserved.

surgical block time, 9 procedures in the ambulatory setting compared with 4 in the hospital OR. A prospective cohort study of 100 procedures done at a military medical center found a cost savings of 85% for CTR and 70% for A1 pulley release compared with the same procedures done in the hospital OR, for a cost savings of approximately $400,000 over 21 months.[10] Nelson and colleagues[11] compared the cost of fasciectomy for Dupuytren contracture in an ambulatory setting to that in a hospital OR and concluded that costs in the OR were 13 times more than in the ambulatory setting. Bismal and colleagues[12] determined that a "one-stop wide-awake hand surgery service" saved the British National Health Service more than $2 million in the past 10 years. Gillis and Williams[13] determined that the use of the hospital OR for closed reduction and internal fixation of hand fractures was associated with a significant increase in costs compared with an ASC, and Mather and colleagues[14] found that volar plating of distal radial fractures overall was 46% less expensive at an ASC than an inpatient facility, regardless of fracture severity, patient age or American Society of Anesthesiologists (ASA) classification, or use of bone graft. Gancarczyk and colleagues[15] reported that open trigger finger release in an ASC was considerably less expensive than in the hospital, and Webb and Stothard[16] reported that outpatient treatment of Dupuytren disease, wrist ganglia, and trigger finger results in substantial cost savings compared with standard surgical treatment in the hospital. They also found that 12 outpatient procedures could be done in the same time period as 3 procedures in a hospital OR.

EFFICIENCY

ASCs often specialize in certain procedures, which leads to increased volume for these specific procedures and leads to improved patient outcomes.[17] By performing more of the same procedure, these centers become more efficient as staff become more familiar with their routines.[18] On average, procedures done in ASCs take 31.8 fewer minutes than those done in hospitals.[18] Gottschalk and colleagues[19] reported that procedures done in an ASC had a turnover time of 27.9 minutes compared with 36.4 minutes in an orthopedic specialty hospital. Hair and colleagues[20] showed, in an analysis of the 2006 National Survey of Ambulatory Surgery public data, that surgical procedures performed in freestanding ASCs took a mean of 39% less total time than those performed in hospital-based ASCs. Chatterjee and colleagues[7] reported more than twice the number of CTS procedures during a 3-hour surgical block time in the ASC, and Goyal and colleagues[6] reported a mean turnover time of 13 minutes in hand and upper extremity surgery at an ASC. High surgeon volume and specialization also are associated with improved patient outcomes.[17]

COMPLICATIONS

Several reports have shown ASC surgery to have a low rate of complications. Goyal and colleagues[6] reviewed 28,737 cases done at an ASC and found only 58 reported adverse events, for an overall rate of 0.2%. In their analysis of 10,646 patients, Lipira and colleagues[21] reported a 2.5% overall frequency of complications within 30 days of surgery; the use of local anesthesia and outpatient surgery (1.4% complication rate) was associated with a significantly lower risk of complications than inpatient surgery (8.7% complication rate). In 14,106 hand and elbow procedures done at more than 450 ASCs over a 2-year period, 169 (1.2%) had unplanned readmissions, most frequently for surgical site infections (0.02% of all procedures).[22] Readmitted patients tended to be 50 years of age or older and were more likely to be smokers; to have diabetes mellitus, hypertension, chronic obstructive pulmonary disease, congestive heart failure, a history of dialysis, dyspnea, and bleeding diatheses; to be on steroids; to have a lower hematocrit, and to have hypoalbuminea. Infections were less frequent in those with local or regional anesthesia (8%) than in those with other types of anesthesia (eg, general, epidural, and spinal) (13%). The study also determined that readmitted patients had more comorbidities and higher ASA levels, leading the investigators to suggest that these patients might be better treated in-hospital by multidisciplinary teams. Munnich and Parente,[23] however, found that the highest-risk Medicare patients were less likely to visit an emergency room or be admitted to a hospital following similar procedures done in an ASC rather than an in-hospital outpatient facility.

Goyal and colleagues[6] reported no wrong-site upper-extremity surgical procedures after 28,737 cases despite hand surgical procedures being high risk for wrong-site surgery.[24,25] Having the attending physician mark the surgical incision site in the preoperative holding area with the patient awake and strictly adhering to a surgical checklist and time out are effective in reducing complications in multiple health care settings.[26] Because most cases are done in less than 1 hour in an ASC, there is less staff hand-over during and after cases, which has been shown to reduce complications.[27]

PATIENT SATISFACTION

In a prospective evaluation of 200 consecutive patients who had hand surgery under general anesthesia in an ASC, 22 patients (11%) were dissatisfied with their experience because of postoperative nausea and vomiting.[28] A nonsmoking history, a history of motion sickness, and a high level of preoperative anxiety were associated with moderate to high levels of nausea and vomiting. The use of local or regional anesthesia or appropriate medications or other intervention should be considered for at-risk patients.[29]

Another reason for patient dissatisfaction is moderate to severe postoperative pain. Inadequate pain management and opioid-related postoperative nausea and vomiting have been cited as leading causes of delayed discharge, unplanned admissions, and patient dissatisfaction.[30] Chung and colleagues[31] reviewed 10,008 consecutive ASC patients with procedures of varying surgical specialties and found that in the recovery room or postanesthesia care unit, orthopedic patients (including those with hand surgery) had the highest frequency of pain. A survey by Rawal and colleagues[32] determined that 37% of hand surgery patients had moderate to severe pain that affected their function and quality of life.

Because of the current concerns about an opioid epidemic, ways to reduce opioid consumption are being investigated. Studies have shown that in general 3 to 5 times more opioids are prescribed than are needed after ASC hand surgery.[33,34] Johnson and colleagues,[35] in a database study of 77,573 opioid-naive patients who had hand surgery, found that 77% filled at least 1 perioperative opioid prescription and 13% continued to fill opioid prescriptions 90 days after surgery. They identified as risk factors for prolonged opioid use younger age, female gender, more comorbid conditions, lower income, mental health disorders and tobacco dependence or abuse. Using insurance claims data from more than 100 US health plans, Waljee and colleagues[36] studied opioid prescriptions in 296,452 adults older than 18 years who had carpal or cubital tunnel release, trigger finger release, or thumb carpometacarpal arthroplasty. They determined that patients who had previously received opioids were more likely to fill a postoperative opioid prescription, receive longer prescription, receive refills after surgery, and have at least 1 indicator of potentially inappropriate prescribing. The probability of filling an opioid prescription declined linearly with advancing age. Dufeu and colleagues[37] described the use of ultrasound-guided distal blocks (along with acetaminophen and nonsteroidal anti-inflammatory drugs and opioids as rescue drugs) in 125 patients with hand or wrist surgery at an ASC. They obtained effective pain control for an average of 12 hours in 96% of patients.

SUMMARY

Outpatient surgery, especially in free-standing ASCs, provides a safe, cost-effective option for a variety of surgical procedures and has become the preferred choice over inpatient and hospital-based outpatient surgery for most hand and wrist procedures. Complication rates after ASC hand surgery are low (0.2%–2.5%), and patient satisfaction is high.

REFERENCES

1. Hall MJ, Schwartzman A, Zhang J, et al. Ambulatory surgery data from hospitals and ambulatory surgery centers: United States, 2010. Natl Health Stat Rep 2017;(102):1–15. Available at: https://www.cdc.gov/nchs/data/nhsr/nhsr102.pdf. Accessed August 15, 2017.
2. Koenig L, Doherty J, Dreyfus J, et al. An analysis of recent growth of ambulatory surgical centers. Final report. 2009. Available at: http://citeseerx.ist.psu.edu/viewdoc/download?doi=10.1.1.512.4498&rep=rep1&type=pdf. Accessed August 15, 2017.
3. Munns JJ, Awan HM. Trends in carpal tunnel surgery: an online survey of members of the American Society for Surgery of the Hand. J Hand Surg Am 2015;40:767–71.
4. Fajardo M, Kim SH, Szabo RM. Incidence of carpal tunnel release: trends and implications with the United States ambulatory care setting. J Hand Surg Am 2012;37(8):1599–605.
5. Patel AA, Buller LT, Fleming ME, et al. National trends in ambulatory surgery for upper extremity fractures: a 10-year analysis of the US National Survey of Ambulatory Surgery. Hand (N Y) 2015;10:254–9.
6. Goyal KS, Jain S, Buterbaugh GA, et al. The safety of hand and upper-extremity surgical procedures at a freestanding ambulatory surgery center: a review of 28,737 cases. J Bone Joint Surg Am 2016;98(8):700–4.
7. Chatterjee A, McCarthy JE, Montagne SA, et al. A cost, profit, and efficiency analysis of performing carpal tunnel surgery in the operating room versus the clinic setting in the United States. Ann Plast Surg 2011;66:245–8.

8. Leblanc MR, Lalonde J, Lalonde DH. A detailed cost and efficiency analysis of performing carpal tunnel surgery in the main operating room versus the ambulatory setting in Canada. Hand (N Y) 2007;2:173–8.

9. Nguyen C, Milstein A, Hernandez-Boussard T, et al. The effect of moving carpal tunnel releases out of hospitals on reducing United States health care charges. J Hand Surg Am 2015;40:1657–62.

10. Rhee PC, Fischer MM, Rhee LS, et al. Cost savings and patient experience of a clinic-based, wide-awake hand surgery program at a military medical center: a critical analysis of the first 100 procedures. J Hand Surg Am 2017;42(3):e139–47.

11. Nelson R, Higgins A, Conrad J, et al. The wide-awake approach to Dupuytren's disease: fasciectomy under local anesthetic with epinephrine. Hand (N Y) 2010;5(2):117–24.

12. Bismil M, Bismil Q, Harding P, et al. Transition to total one-stop wide-awake hand surgery service-audit: a retrospective review. JRSM Short Rep 2012;3(4):23.

13. Gillis JA, Williams JG. Cost analysis of percutaneous fixation of hand fractures in the main operating room versus the ambulatory setting. J Plast Reconstr Aesthet Surg 2017;70(8):1044–50.

14. Mather RC 3rd, Wysocki RW, Mack Aldridge J 3rd, et al. Effect of facility on the operative costs of distal radius fractures. J Hand Surg Am 2011;36(7):1142–8.

15. Gancarczyk SM, Jang ES, Swart EP, et al. Percutaneous trigger finger release: a cost-effectiveness analysis. J Am Acad Orthop Surg 2016;24(7):475–82.

16. Webb JA, Stothard J. Cost minimization using clinic-based treatment for common hand conditions—a prospective economic analysis. Ann R Coll Surg Engl 2009;91:135–9.

17. Chowdjury MM, Dagash H, Pierro A. A systematic review of the impact of volume of surgery and specialization on patient outcome. Br J Surg 2007; 94(2):145–61.

18. Munnich EL, Parente ST. Procedures take less time at ambulatory surgery centers, keeping costs down and ability to meet demand up. Health Aff (Millwood) 2014;35(5):764–9.

19. Gottschalk MD, Hinds RM, Muppavarapu TC, et al. Factors affecting hand surgeon operating room turnover time. Hand (N Y) 2016;11(4):489–94.

20. Hair B, Hussey P, Wynn B. A comparison of ambulatory perioperative times in hospitals and free-standing centers. Am J Surg 2012;204:23–7.

21. Lipira AB, Sood RF, Tatman PD, et al. Complications within 30 days of hand surgery: an analysis of 10,646 patients. J Hand Surg Am 2015;40(9):1952–9.

22. Noureldin M, Habermann EB, Ubl DS, et al. Unplanned readmissions following outpatient hand

and elbow surgery. J Bone Joint Surg Am 2017; 99(7):541–9.

23. Munnich EL, Parente ST. Procedures take less time at ambulatory surgery centers, keeping costs down and ability to meet demand up. Health Aff (Millwood) 2014;33(5):764–9.

24. Meinberg EG, Stern PJ. Incidence of wrong-site surgery among hand surgeons. J Bone Joint Surg Am 2003;85(2):193–7.

25. Robinson PM, Muir LT. Wrong-site surgery in orthopaedics. J Bone Joint Surg Br 2009;91(10):1274–80.

26. Weiser TG, Haynes AB, Lashoher A, et al. Perspectives in quality: designing the WHO surgical safety checklist. Int J Qual Health Care 2010;22(5):365–70.

27. Smith AF, Pope C, Goodwin D, et al. Interprofessional handover and patient safety in anaesthesia: observational study of handovers in the recovery room. Br J Anaesth 2008;101(3):332–7.

28. Roh YH, Gong HS, Kim JH, et al. Factors associated with postoperative nausea and vomiting in patients undergoind an ambulatory hand surgery. Clin Orthop Surg 2014;6(3):273–8.

29. Geralemou S, Gan TI. Assessing the value of risk indices of postoperative nausea and vomiting in ambulatory surgical patients. Curr Opin Anaesthesiol 2016;29(6):668–73.

30. Rodgers J, Cunningham K, Fitzgerald K, et al. Opioid consumption following outpatient upper extremity surgery. J Hand Surg Am 2012;37(4):645–50.

31. Chung F, Ritchie E, Su J. Postoperative pain in ambulatory surgery. Anesth Analg 1997;85(4):808–16.

32. Rawal N, Hylander J, Nydahl PA, et al. Survey of postoperative analgesia following ambulatory surgery. Acta Anaesthesiol Scand 1997;41(8):1017–22.

33. Chapman T, Kim N, Maltenfort M, et al. Prospective evaluation of opioid consumption following carpal tunnel release surgery. Hand (N Y) 2017;12(1):39–42.

34. Kim N, Matzon JL, Abboudi J, et al. A prospective evaluation of opioid utilization after upper-extremity surgical procedures: identifying consumption patterns and determining prescribing guidelines. J Bone Joint Surg Am 2016;98(20):e89.

35. Johnson SP, Chung KC, Zhong L, et al. Risk of prolonged opioid use among opioid-naïve patients following common hand surgery procedures. J Hand Surg Am 2016;41(10):947–57.

36. Waljee JF, Zhong L, Hou H, et al. The use of opioid analgesics following common upper extremity surgical procedures: a national, population-based study. Plast Reconstr Surg 2016;137(2):355e–64e.

37. Dufeu N, Marchard-Maillet F, Atchabahian A, et al. Efficacy and safety of ultrasound-guided distal blocks for analgesia without motor blockade after ambulatory hand surgery. J Hand Surg Am 2014; 39(4):737–43.

Shoulder and Elbow

Outpatient Shoulder Arthroplasty

Tyler J. Brolin, MD, Thomas W. Throckmorton, MD*

KEYWORDS

- Ambulatory surgery center • Outpatient • Shoulder arthroplasty • Joint replacement
- Cost-effectiveness • Outcomes • Complications • Readmission rate

KEY POINTS

- Outpatient shoulder arthroplasty seems to be a safe alternative to shoulder arthroplasty performed in a traditional inpatient setting in appropriately selected patients.
- Appropriate patient selection, multimodal pain management strategies, minimizing blood loss, and efficient operative times are paramount to successful outpatient shoulder arthroplasty.
- Shoulder arthroplasties performed in an outpatient setting may offer significant cost savings compared with those performed in an inpatient hospital setting.

INTRODUCTION

The demand for shoulder arthroplasty continues to see tremendous growth. With a procedure volume growth rate of 9.4% per year, total shoulder arthroplasty (TSA) demand is increasing at a rate surpassing that of lower-extremity arthroplasty.[1] This substantial increase is likely due to multiple factors, including an aging patient population, improved implant design, the expanded role of reverse TSA, and improvements in perioperative pain management. The increased number of TSA procedures being performed each year translates to increased health care–related expenditures. As health care policy continues to evolve, now more than ever, the emphasis has been placed on providing safe, high-quality health care in an efficient and cost-effective manner. Recently, bundled payment programs have been initiated to help control the costs associated with total joint arthroplasty. These programs place increased financial responsibility on the surgeon

to control 90-day episode-of-care costs, including limiting or eliminating reimbursement for early complications or readmissions. This increased responsibility underscores the important balance surgeons face today in implementing cost-saving measures without jeopardizing outcomes or safety. One particular area of cost savings is transitioning total joint arthroplasties (TJAs) from a traditional inpatient setting to an outpatient setting for selected patients.

TJA has traditionally remained an inpatient procedure because of concerns over pain control, blood loss, and potential postoperative complications. These factors underscore the key steps in the transition to outpatient TSA (Fig. 1). Overall, improved surgical techniques, pain management, and perioperative patient management have led to declining lengths of stay. A study of 2004 patients who had a TSA from 2005 to 2011 found the average length of stay after TSA was 2.2 days.[2] Today, many patients can be discharged after one night in

Disclosure Statement: T.J. Brolin: no disclosures. T.W. Throckmorton: IP royalties, Zimmer Biomet; speaker, Zimmer Biomet; consultant, Zimmer Biomet; stock/stock options, Gilead; research support, Zimmer Biomet; publishing royalties, Elsevier.

Shoulder and Elbow Surgery, Department of Orthopaedic Surgery, University of Tennessee-Campbell Clinic, 1211 Union Avenue, Suite 510, Memphis, TN 38104, USA

* Corresponding author.

E-mail address: tthrockmorton@campbellclinic.com

Orthop Clin N Am 49 (2018) 73–79
http://dx.doi.org/10.1016/j.ocl.2017.08.011

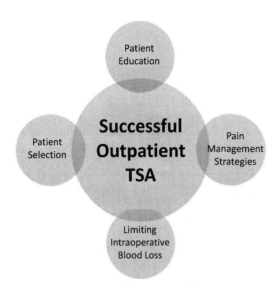

Fig. 1. Keys to successful outpatient TSA.

the hospital. In a recent series of 30 patients who had TSA in the traditional inpatient hospital setting, the average length of stay was 1.1 days[3]; in a survey of American Shoulder and Elbow Surgeons members, 69.8% of shoulder surgeons responded that their patients had an average length of stay of less than 1.5 days (unpublished data Brolin, June 2017). In the authors' experience, most patients who have inpatient shoulder arthroplasty spend a night in the hospital and are discharged the following day. This practice has led to a natural transition to performing TSAs in the ambulatory setting when possible.

PATIENT SELECTION

One of the main concerns regarding outpatient TJA is whether potential complications will occur and lead to increased morbidity and hospital readmission. This concern has been refuted by multiple reports that have documented the success of outpatient lower extremity arthroplasty without jeopardizing patient safety or satisfaction.[4–7] Nelson and colleagues[6] recently reported their findings using the National Surgical Quality Improvement Program (NSQIP) database to identify 63,844 patients who had total hip arthroplasties (THAs). They compared those patients who had THA as an outpatient with those whose hospital stays were 1 to 5 days. There were no differences in any of the 18 adverse events they evaluated except for the need for a blood transfusion, which was significantly less in the outpatient cohort.

The rates of complications, mortality, and readmission compare favorably for TSA compared with THA and total knee arthroplasty (TKA).[8,9] An analysis of 15,414 THAs, 34,471 TKAs, and 994 TSAs done between 2000 and 2009 showed significantly lower mortality and complication rates for TSA than for THA and TKA.[8] The inpatient complication rate for TSA was 7.6% compared with 14.7% for TKA and 15.5% for THA. This analysis was followed up with a study using the Veterans Administration's National Surgical Quality Improvement Program database from 1999 to 2006, which showed that the 30-day mortality rates were 1.2%, 1.1%, and 0.4% for THA, TKA, and TSA, respectively.[9] Patients with TSA had a 30-day complication rate of 2.8%, compared with 7.6% for THA and 6.8% for TKA. This comparative complication profile has also led to increased interest in transitioning TSA to an outpatient procedure.

The recently published rates of early complications after TSA range from 2.8% to 9.4%.[8–13] Although these are relatively low rates of complications, a complication in an ambulatory surgery center (ASC) environment could potentially be catastrophic. Courtney and colleagues[14] had an important study examining which patients should not undergo short-stay THA and TKA. Their retrospective review of 1012 patients reported an overall complication rate of 6.9%. Of those complications that required physician intervention, 84% occurred more than 24 hours postoperatively. Multivariate analysis concluded that patients with chronic obstructive pulmonary disease (COPD), coronary artery disease (CAD), congestive heart failure (CHF), and cirrhosis had a significantly increased risk of complications. This finding led the investigators to strongly advocate against these patients undergoing outpatient arthroplasty. This experience underlines the importance of proper medical evaluation preoperatively to identify patient factors that put them at an increased risk of a complication or readmission after joint arthroplasty. Also, because a significant proportion of TJAs require only a 1-night stay in the hospital, most complications will occur after discharge regardless of the operative setting.

Several recent studies have examined potential risk factors for morbidity, mortality, and readmission after TSA (Box 1). These studies are critical in our understanding of which patients are eligible for outpatient TSA after appropriate preoperative medical and anesthesia evaluations. Two studies examined the risk factors associated with 30-day morbidity. Anthony and colleagues[10] found that having a

Box 1
Risk factors for complications or hospital readmissions following shoulder arthroplasty

- Increased number of comorbidities (ASA class 4)
- Coronary artery disease
- Congestive heart failure
- Peripheral vascular disease
- Chronic obstructive pulmonary disease
- Anemia (hematocrit <38)
- Cirrhosis
- Obesity
- Increased operative time (>2 hours)

Abbreviation: ASA, American Society of Anesthesiologists.

complication within the first 30 days was associated with chronic steroid use, a preoperative hematocrit of less than 38%, American Society of Anesthesiologists (ASA) class 4, and an operative time longer than 2 hours. A history of CHF was also associated with an increased mortality rate. Waterman and colleagues[12] also found preexisting cardiac disease to be a significant risk factor. Both cardiac disease and increased age were associated with a higher risk of mortality, and both peripheral vascular disease (PVD) and operative time of more than 174 minutes were associated with increased complications. Two other studies extended the postoperative follow-up period to 90 days and found that higher Charlson Comorbidity Index (CCI), PVD, and performing TSA for a proximal humeral fracture were related to increased complications.[11,13] Some of the most devastating complications are cardiopulmonary, which fortunately are infrequent after TSA whereby the risk of a 90-day cardiac or venous thromboembolic event is 2.6% and 1.2%, respectively.[15] Finally, increased age, comorbidities, and prior cardiac events are related to an increased probability of a postoperative cardiac event.

It is imperative that the surgeon be comfortable with TSA before performing outpatient TSA. As the previously mentioned studies have shown, increased operative time increases the complication rate following TSA.[10,12] Therefore, it is important to perform the procedure efficiently to avoid unnecessary complications and minimize blood loss. Also, from a logistical standpoint, ASCs have limited implants and instruments available to safely, efficiently, and reproducibly perform TSA.

Readmission after TJA is a major concern, not only for the obvious reason of putting the safety and well-being of the patient at risk but it also leads to increased episode-of-care costs and consumes health care resources. Unplanned readmissions are being increasingly scrutinized and may not be reimbursed in bundled payment programs. The 90-day readmission rates after TSA range from 2.5% to 6.6%.[16–19] Age, increased comorbidities, and obesity have been shown to be factors increasing the rate of readmission. It may be intuitive that an increasing number of comorbid conditions puts patients at risk of complication or readmission, but relying on just the ASA score or CCI may not be sufficient in predicting successful outpatient TJA. Meneghini and colleagues[20] established the Outpatient Arthroplasty Risk Assessment Score (OARA), which is composed of 9 comorbid areas, all weighted differently in importance, to screen patients for THA. They used an OARA score of 59 or less as the cutoff and found that this had a positive predictive value of 81.6 for early discharge, with a 90-day rehospitalization rate of 2.9%, and it outperformed the ASA and CCI. As TSA transitions to being performed at freestanding ASCs, the ability to predict which patients can be discharged on the day of surgery is critical. Unplanned overnight stays or transfers to a hospital increase episode-of-care costs after TJA as well as strain the ASC facility and personnel who have to deliver health care overnight.

Another concern regarding TJA is the need for postoperative blood transfusion. Padegimas and colleagues[21] retrospectively reviewed 1174 TSAs and the overall rate of blood transfusion was 4.5%. They found that predictors of receiving a blood transfusion were lower preoperative hematocrit levels and posttraumatic arthritis as an operative indication. A preoperative hematocrit of less than 39.6% resulted in an 11.0% chance of receiving a blood transfusion compared with 0.7% with a level greater than that threshold. Preoperative laboratory values with specific attention to hematocrit and hemoglobin levels are an important part of the screening process for outpatient TSA. Recently, the use of tranexamic acid has been advocated to reduce blood loss and transfusion need after TSA although the authors have no experience with using tranexamic acid, this may prove a useful adjunct to preventing transfusions, especially in higher-risk patients.[22–25]

PERIOPERATIVE PAIN MANAGEMENT

Advances in perioperative patient management, most notably improvements in pain management techniques, have made the transition of TSA to an ambulatory procedure possible. In the past, postoperative pain regimens consisted of oral and intravenous narcotics, usually with a patient-controlled anesthesia pump. There has been a paradigm shift that stresses limiting narcotic use and focusing on multiple modalities for pain control. A multimodal pain management program using long- and short-acting narcotics and antiinflammatories as well as neuroleptic agents, such as gabapentin or pregabalin given immediately before and after surgery, has been used with success.[26] These medications can be given in conjunction with regional anesthesia in the form of an interscalene nerve block or an intraoperative periarticular injection with bupivacaine.

Currently, there is much debate regarding the ideal form of pain management, and most of this has surrounded the use of an interscalene nerve block versus liposomal bupivacaine. Recently, there have been 3 high-quality studies comparing liposomal bupivacaine and interscalene blockade.[27–29] Weller and colleagues[27] compared 156 patients who received interscalene catheters with 58 patients who received liposomal bupivacaine after TSA. They found no difference in the visual analogue scores at 24 hours, 2 weeks, 6 weeks, or 12 weeks; the interscalene catheter group had significantly more major complications. Namdari and colleagues[28] conducted a randomized controlled trial comparing liposomal bupivacaine and interscalene nerve blocks. The patients receiving interscalene blocks had significantly less pain at 8 hours postoperatively but had significantly more pain at 24 hours, likely due to rebound pain. This finding was also seen in the study by Okoroha and colleagues,[29] whereby patients receiving interscalene nerve blocks required more opioids at postoperative hours 13 through 16 and on postoperative day zero overall but had significantly better pain relief for the first 8 hours. Whether the surgeon chooses a periarticular injection or regional anesthesia is likely institutionally dependent along with the degree of comfort with the anesthesia team. Both seem to be a better alternative to narcotics alone, but further research is needed. What is clear, however, is that a pain management strategy that uses multiple modalities and focuses on blocking multiple pain pathways is key to reliable discharge following outpatient TJA and is of paramount importance to a successful outpatient TJA program.

SAFETY OF OUTPATIENT SHOULDER ARTHROPLASTY

The emergence of outpatient TSA has lagged behind that of lower extremity arthroplasty performed in an ambulatory setting. Currently, there are just 3 studies that have examined the complication and readmission rates after outpatient TSA.[3,30,31] Leroux and colleagues[30] performed a retrospective cohort study using the ACS NSQIP, which gathers all patient-specific characteristics as well as data on adverse events and readmissions within the first 30 days postoperatively. A total of 7197 patients who had primary total TSA were identified, including 173 (2.4%) who had outpatient TSA. Outpatients were defined as a length of stay of 0 days, whereas inpatients were defined as a length of stay greater than 0 days. Overall, the outpatient cohort had 4 patients who had adverse events (2.3%), no deaths, and 2 readmissions (1.9%). Important to note was the significant selection bias, as the outpatients were significantly younger, had a lower body mass index (BMI), and lower ASA scores. The investigators found that the odds of an adverse event or readmission were not significantly different between the two groups.

Another database study from Cancienne and colleagues[31] used the PearlDiver database to compare the rates of readmission and adverse events between patients with inpatient and outpatient TSA. The patients with outpatient TSA were identified by service location first and were confirmed to have a length of stay of 0 days and no inpatient codes. A total of 703 ambulatory TSAs were matched to 4459 inpatient TSAs. The incidence of outpatient TSAs increased by 107% from 2011 to 2014. The overall 90-day complication and readmission rates for the outpatient cohort were 15.9% and 9.3%, respectively. There was no significant difference in complication rate or readmission rate between groups, although the chance of receiving a blood transfusion or having a urinary tract infection was increased in the inpatient cohort. Medically related readmissions represented 81.8% of all readmissions in the ambulatory group. Significant risk factors for readmission after outpatient TSAs were obesity, diabetes, PVD, CHF, depression, chronic anemia, and chronic lung disease.

Finally, the authors compared 30 outpatient TSAs at a freestanding ASC with an age- and comorbidities-matched cohort of 30 patients who had traditional inpatient TSAs.[3] It is important to note that these patients had true outpatient TSAs, as they were discharged on the day of surgery with no overnight stays, the latter of which may represent part of the outpatient cohorts in the database studies. Ninety-day episode-of-care complications, including hospital admissions or readmissions, and reoperations were evaluated. There were no differences in age, ASA score, BMI, or operative indications between the groups. Importantly, there were no cardiopulmonary complications, mortalities, or admissions in the outpatient group. Overall, the complication rates were not significantly different.

COST-EFFECTIVENESS OF OUTPATIENT SHOULDER ARTHROPLASTY

The health care system continues to become increasingly cognizant of costs of care. Ways to decrease cost without jeopardizing patient safety or clinical outcomes remain a challenge. One avenue is the transition of patients with TJAs into the outpatient setting, thus, eliminating unnecessary costs associated with routine hospital admission. With the number of TJAs performed each year continuing to increase at a significant rate, eliminating unnecessary health care expenditures could translate to significant cost savings to the health care system. Recently, there have been a few reports evaluating outpatient TJA as a means of cost reduction.

Lovald and colleagues[32] compared the 2-year costs associated with outpatient and inpatient TKA. The 2-year costs associated with the outpatient TKA group were $8527 less than that of the group staying 3 to 4 days after TKA. Another study by Aynardi and colleagues[33] found that the average costs associated with outpatient THA were $24,529, compared with $31,327 for inpatient THA, for an overall savings of $6798. Cancienne and colleagues[31] found the drug related group (DRG)-related costs were significantly lower for ambulatory TSAs compared with inpatient TSAs, with total costs of $14,722 and $18,336, respectively. Although long-term outcome studies evaluating outpatient TSA are lacking, it seems that outpatient TSA is a safe and cost-effective alternative to inpatient TSA in appropriately selected patients.

AUTHORS' EXPERIENCE WITH OUTPATIENT TOTAL SHOULDER ARTHROPLASTY

At the authors' institution, potential outpatient TSA candidates are first screened by the surgeon based on several criteria, including the patients' wishes, social situation, and overall health status. During the preoperative office visit, a thorough discussion is held with patients regarding the authors' outpatient process and reasonable expectations. Patients then undergo a preanesthetic evaluation at the ASC under the supervision of a staff anesthesiologist familiar with outpatient joint arthroplasty. The evaluation includes a review of the patients' health history and medications, with special attention to pulmonary and cardiac morbidities. A preoperative hematocrit of less than 30% is a contraindication for outpatient TSA because of the increased risk for blood transfusion; these patients are sent for an anemia workup and reevaluated on completion of the workup. Significant pulmonary comorbidities and high risk after cardiology consultation also are contraindications for outpatient TSA.

A multimodal pain management program is used, including long- and short-acting oral oxycodone, acetaminophen, and gabapentin, unless contraindicated. These medications are given immediately before and after surgery. Intraoperatively, a periarticular injection consisting of liposomal bupivacaine, bupivacaine, and ketorolac is placed in the deltoid, pectoralis major, and subcutaneous tissues surrounding the incision. After surgery, patients are evaluated in the postanesthesia care unit. Once pain is adequately controlled and patients are able to urinate and ambulate without assistance, they are discharged home. The following day, a staff member of the ASC calls patients to answer any questions and ensure adequate pain control. The first postoperative clinic visit occurs approximately 14 days following the procedure. Using this protocol, all patients have been able to be discharged from the ASC on the day of surgery with no cardiopulmonary complications that required hospital admission or intervention.

SUMMARY

The health care environment is evolving, and surgeons are under increasing pressure to deliver high-quality health care that is efficient and cost-effective. This requirement, however, must not come at a cost to patient safety or clinical outcomes. The literature thus far has supported outpatient TSA as a safe and cost-effective alternative to routine hospital admission. Proper patient selection is of paramount importance to prevent complications and hospital admissions. Advances in pain control techniques, most notably multimodal pain management programs, regional anesthesia, and liposomal bupivacaine, have been key in the evolution of outpatient TSA programs.

REFERENCES

1. Day JS, Lau E, Ong KL, et al. Prevalence and projections of total shoulder and elbow arthroplasty in the United States to 2015. J Shoulder Elbow Surg 2010;19:1115–20.
2. Dunn JC, Lanzi J, Kusnezov N, et al. Predictors of length of stay after elective total shoulder arthroplasty in the United States. J Shoulder Elbow Surg 2015;24:754–9.
3. Brolin TJ, Mulligan RP, Azar FM, et al. Neer award 2016: outpatient total shoulder arthroplasty in an ambulatory surgery center is a safe alternative to inpatient total shoulder arthroplasty in a hospital: a matched cohort study. J Shoulder Elbow Surg 2017;26:204–8.
4. Berger RA, Kusuma SK, Sanders SA, et al. The feasibility and perioperative complications of outpatient knee arthroplasty. Clin Orthop Relat Res 2009; 467(6):1443–9.
5. Berger RA, Sanders S, Gerlinger T, et al. Outpatient total knee arthroplasty with a minimally invasive technique. J Arthroplasty 2005;20(7 Suppl 3):33–8.
6. Nelson SJ, Webb ML, Lukasiewicz AM, et al. Is outpatient total hip arthroplasty safe? J Arthroplasty 2017;32:1439–42.
7. Kolisek FR, McGrath MS, Jessup NM, et al. Comparison of outpatient versus inpatient total knee arthroplasty. Clin Orthop Relat Res 2009;467: 1438–42.
8. Farmer KW, Hammond JW, Queale WS, et al. Shoulder arthroplasty versus hip and knee arthroplasties: a comparison of outcomes. Clin Orthop Relat Res 2007;455:183–9.
9. Fehringer EV, Mikuls TR, Michaud KD, et al. Shoulder arthroplasties have fewer complications than hip or knee arthroplasties in US veterans. Clin Orthop Relat Res 2010;468:717–22.
10. Anthony CA, Westermann RW, Gao Y, et al. What are risk factors for 30-day morbidity and transfusion in total shoulder arthroplasty? A review of 1922 cases. Clin Orthop Relat Res 2015;473:2099–105.
11. Farng E, Zingmond D, Krenek L, et al. Factors predicting complication rates after primary shoulder arthroplasty. J Shoulder Elbow Surg 2011;20: 557–63.
12. Waterman BR, Dunn JC, Bader J, et al. Thirty-day morbidity and mortality after elective total shoulder arthroplasty: patient-based and surgical risk factors. J Shoulder Elbow Surg 2015;24:24–30.
13. Chalmers PN, Gupta AK, Rahman Z, et al. Predictors of early complications of total shoulder arthroplasty. J Arthroplasty 2014;29:856–60.
14. Courtney PM, Rozell JC, Melnic CM, et al. Who should not undergo short stay hip and knee arthroplasty? Risk factors associated with major medical complications following primary total joint arthroplasty. J Arthroplasty 2015;30(9 Suppl):1–4.
15. Singh JA, Sperling JW, Cofield RH. Cardiopulmonary complications after primary shoulder arthroplasty: a cohort study. Semin Arthritis Rheum 2012;41:689–97.
16. Matsen FA, Li N, Gao H, et al. Factors affecting length of stay, readmission, and revision after shoulder arthroplasty: a population-based study. J Bone Joint Surg Am 2015;97:1255–63.
17. Mahoney A, Bosco JA, Zuckerman JD. Readmission after shoulder arthroplasty. J Shoulder Elbow Surg 2014;23:377–81.
18. Anakwenze O, Fokin A, Chocas M, et al. Complications in total shoulder and reverse total shoulder arthroplasty by body mass index. J Shoulder Elbow Surg 2017;26(7):1230–7.
19. Westermann RW, Anthony CA, Duchman KR, et al. Incidence, causes and predictors of 30-day readmission after shoulder arthroplasty. Iowa Orthop J 2016;36:70–4.
20. Meneghini RM, Ziemba-Davis M, Ishmael MK, et al. Safe selection of outpatient joint arthroplasty patients with medical risk stratification: the "outpatient arthroplasty risk assessment score". J Arthroplasty 2017; 32(8):2325–31.
21. Padegimas EM, Clyde CT, Zmistowski BM, et al. Risk factors for blood transfusion after shoulder arthroplasty. Bone Joint J 2016;98-B:224–8.
22. Abildgaard JT, McLemore R, Hattrup SJ. Tranexamic acid decreases blood loss in total shoulder arthroplasty and reverse total shoulder arthroplasty. J Shoulder Elbow Surg 2016;25:1643–8.
23. Vara AD, Koueiter DM, Pinkas DE, et al. Intravenous tranexamic acid reduces total blood loss in reverse total shoulder arthroplasty: a prospective, double-blinded, randomized, controlled trial. J Shoulder Elbow Surg 2017;26(8):1383–9.
24. Friedman RJ, Gordon E, Butler RB, et al. Tranexamic acid decreases blood loss after total shoulder arthroplasty. J Shoulder Elbow Surg 2016;25:614–8.
25. Gillespie R, Shishani Y, Joseph S, et al. Neer award 2015: a randomized, prospective evaluation on the effectiveness of tranexamic acid in reducing blood loss after total shoulder arthroplasty. J Shoulder Elbow Surg 2015;24:1679–84.
26. Warrender WJ, Syed UAM, Hammoud S, et al. Pain management after outpatient shoulder arthroscopy: a systematic review of randomized controlled trials. Am J Sports Med 2017;45(7):1676–86.
27. Weller WJ, Azzam MG, Smith RA, et al. Liposomal bupivacaine mixture has similar pain relief and significantly fewer complications at less cost compared to indwelling interscalene catheter in

total shoulder arthroplasty. J Arthroplasty 2017. Epub ahead of print.

28. Namdari S, Nicholson T, Abboud J, et al. Randomized controlled trial of interscalene block compared with injectable liposomal bupivacaine in shoulder arthroplasty. J Bone Joint Surg Am 2017;99:550–6.

29. Okoroha KR, Lynch JR, Keller RA, et al. Liposomal bupivacaine versus interscalene nerve block for pain control after shoulder arthroplasty: a prospective randomized trial. J Shoulder Elbow Surg 2016; 25:1742–8.

30. Leroux TS, Basques BA, Frank RM, et al. Outpatient total shoulder arthroplasty: a population-based study comparing adverse event and readmission rates to inpatient total shoulder arthroplasty. J Shoulder Elbow Surg 2016;25:1780–6.

31. Cancienne JM, Brockmeier SF, Gulotta LV, et al. Ambulatory total shoulder arthroplasty: a comprehensive analysis of current trends, complications, readmissions, and costs. J Bone Joint Surg Am 2017;99:629–37.

32. Lovald ST, Ong KL, Malkani AL, et al. Complications, mortality, and costs for outpatient and short-stay total knee arthroplasty patients in comparison to standard-stay patients. J Arthroplasty 2014;29:510–5.

33. Aynardi M, Post Z, Ong A, et al. Outpatient surgery as a means of cost reduction in total hip arthroplasty: a case-control study. HSS J 2014;10:252–5.

Pain Management Strategies in Shoulder Arthroplasty

Jason L. Codding, MD*, Charles L. Getz, MD

KEYWORDS

- Multimodal analgesia • Shoulder arthroplasty • Outpatient surgery • Pain control
- Open shoulder surgery • Opioid • Regional anesthesia

KEY POINTS

- Pain control in total shoulder arthroplasty demands a multidisciplinary approach with collaboration between the patients, surgeon, and anesthetist.
- A multimodal approach with preemptive medication, regional blockade, local anesthetics, and a combination of acetaminophen, nonsteroidal antiinflammatory drugs, tramadol, and gabapentinoids postoperatively leads to excellent pain control and patient satisfaction.
- Assessment of patients' expectations constitutes a vital aspect of the preoperative patient evaluation. Educating and psychologically preparing patients reduces postoperative pain.
- Patients with anxiety and depression, preoperative narcotic use, and medical comorbidities are at an increased risk for less effective pain control.
- Minimizing narcotic use decreases opioid-related adverse effects and facilitates productive rehabilitation efforts.

POSTOPERATIVE PAIN IN ORTHOPEDIC AND SHOULDER SURGERY

Shoulder arthroplasty has become a popular definitive treatment option for painful end-stage glenohumeral arthritis, and the demand for arthroplasty surgery is increasing.[1] Although shoulder arthroplasty provides durable long-term clinical results and lasting pain relief,[2–4] early postoperative pain is a major concern following orthopedic surgery and it is an unfavorable outcome causing distress to patients.[5,6] Shoulder surgery has the potential to cause significant postoperative pain, which often necessitates opioid medication.[7] Although opioids are effective in relieving postoperative pain at rest, 70% of patients reported severe pain on movement after open major shoulder and knee surgery.[6] Adequate control of pain is, therefore, critical to facilitate early rehabilitation. Opioid-only analgesic regimens for shoulder surgery are commonly associated with opioid-related adverse effects. These effects include nausea and vomiting, respiratory depression, somnolence, pruritus, sleep disturbances, urinary retention, constipation, and tolerance and may interfere with productive rehabilitation efforts postoperatively.[7–11]

Single analgesics alone are not able to provide adequate pain relief for most moderate or severe pain.[5,12] The dependence solely on opioid medication and the subsequent long-term adverse effects of inadequate pain control have been well described. These consequences include nociception-induced central sensitization and opioid-induced secondary hyperalgesia.

Disclosure Statement: The authors did not receive any outside funding or grants in support of their research for or preparation of this work.

The Rothman Institute at Thomas Jefferson University, Department of Orthopaedic Surgery, 925 Chestnut Street, 5th floor, Philadelphia, PA 19107, USA

* Corresponding author. 1025 Walnut Street Suite 516 College Building, Philadelphia, PA 19107.

E-mail address: jasoncodding@gmail.com

Both of these mechanisms may be involved in the pathogenesis of persistent postsurgical pain.[7,13,14]

The Multimodal Approach

Recognizing the limitations of single analgesic pain regimens has led to the development of alternative strategies for analgesia. A combined approach, known as multimodal analgesia, achieves success by using the additive or synergistic effects between analgesics of different mechanisms and is currently recommended for effective postoperative pain control.[5,15] This approach results in a reduction of side effects from the resulting lower total doses of analgesics and differences in side effect profiles.[15]

The use of multimodal analgesia decreases pain scores and the requirement for postoperative analgesics in a variety of surgical procedures.[5] In one study, a multimodal analgesia clinical pathway evaluated for total shoulder arthroplasty provided excellent results and low pain scores, with half of the patients using little or no intravenous opiates.[16] Additionally, patients undergoing total hip or total knee arthroplasty using a comprehensive, preemptive, multimodal analgesia regimen emphasizing a peripheral nerve blockade have improved perioperative outcomes and fewer adverse events.[17]

The multimodal approach frequently incorporates regional blockade, local anesthetics, and a combination of acetaminophen, nonsteroidal antiinflammatory medications (NSAIDs), tramadol, and gabapentinoids postoperatively to reduce opioid consumption.[7] Regional blockade combats pain transmission through the central nervous system, whereas local anesthetics block sympathetic efferents and axon reflex to decrease pain transmission from tissue.[18] NSAIDs reduce prostaglandin synthesis and inhibit the initiation of pain signals through peripheral blockade of cyclooxygenase (COX) pathways.[19–21] Opioids act on specific opioid receptors in the central nervous system to attenuate pain-related signals,[20] whereas gabapentinoids are lipophilic gamma-aminobutyric acid (GABA) analogues shown to be effective in neuropathic pain, incisional injury, and inflammatory injury.[22]

Medication given before the start of a procedure is known as preemptive analgesia. Preemptive analgesia seeks to prevent hypersensitivity by blocking sensory inputs that induce central sensitization caused by inflammatory injury.[23] Acetaminophen, NSAIDs, and gabapentinoids given to patients in the immediate preoperative period has been investigated.[24–27]

These studies have demonstrated reduced postoperative pain and reduced opioid consumption when given preoperatively.

PREOPERATIVE PATIENT CONSIDERATIONS

Patient Expectations

Optimal postoperative analgesia includes an evaluation of patients' postoperative expectations. Patients undergoing a variety of shoulder procedures have multiple expectations of surgery that vary by diagnosis, age, demographic characteristics, and functional status.[28,29] Outcome expectation plays a significant role in symptom improvement for a variety of shoulder-related complaints, and higher outcome expectations are associated with greater perceived improvements in shoulder function.[30] In a systematic review of 16 moderate-quality evidence articles analyzing the relation between expectations and outcomes, 15 showed positive expectations were associated with better health outcomes.[31] In patients undergoing rotator cuff repair, patients' preoperative expectations were associated with actual self-assessed outcome.[32] Expectations were a significant independent predictor of better outcome scores.

Preoperative educational classes can modify patients' preoperative expectations of their recovery from arthroplasty.[33] Furthermore, psychological preparation for patients has been shown to reduce the need for postoperative analgesics.[34] Carefully presented information from surgeons, anesthetists, and nurses about the procedure, anticipated sensory experiences, analgesic treatment, and recovery period is expected to reduce anxiety.

Anxiety and Depression

Studies investigating depression and anxiety show that preoperative psychological status may negatively influence postoperative outcome and is an essential part of the preoperative assessment.[35] Depression is present in 12.4% of patients undergoing total shoulder arthroplasty; it is twice as common in women, more prevalent in the low-income and Medicaid population, and often underdiagnosed.[36] Postoperative symptoms of distress and depression are associated with worse perceived improvement of pain.[37] As the perception of pain increases, greater opioid analgesic requirements can contribute to postoperative delirium; therefore, depression has been identified as an independent risk factor for postoperative delirium.[36] Depressive symptoms strongly influence perceived disability due to shoulder pain that becomes chronic in nature, and a depressed mood is a useful predictor of surgical outcome when assessing continued pain.[38,39]

Preoperative Narcotic Use

The use of opioid medication as a nonoperative treatment modality for chronic musculoskeletal pain is increasing.[40] Preoperative identification of patients taking opioid medication for pain constitutes an important step in the treatment of postoperative pain. Preoperative opioid history is associated with significantly lower preoperative and postoperative patient-reported outcome measurements compared with an opioid-naïve group in patients undergoing anatomic and reverse total shoulder arthroplasty.[41,42] Additionally, fewer patients in the opioid group were satisfied after surgery.[42] Preoperative opioid history is associated with a lower baseline functional score, and these patients should not be expected to reach the same peak outcome scores after shoulder arthroplasty as those without a preoperative opioid history.[41,42]

Worse clinical outcomes in patients with a preoperative opioid history have been described in other orthopedic subspecialties, including spine surgery and total knee arthroplasty.[43–45] Preoperative opioid use is associated with a longer duration of postoperative opioid use and postoperative doctor shopping.[43,46–48]

Medical Comorbidity

Patients with a greater number of comorbidities have significantly more shoulder pain, worse function, and worse general health status.[49] Although comorbidities are often difficult to modify, postoperative morbidity is related to preoperative comorbidity. Assessment of risks preoperatively and implementation of the treatment of medical optimization are essential.[34]

REGIONAL ANESTHESIA

Regional anesthesia has increased in popularity in shoulder arthroplasty as a means of providing postoperative analgesia. Techniques have been developed to help manage the dynamic pain of shoulder surgery, which include interscalene brachial plexus block, suprascapular nerve block, and supraclavicular nerve block.[11] Increasing the use of ultrasound imaging has facilitated the advancement of these techniques, providing accurate identification of the brachial plexus and its branches.

The brachial plexus supplies all of the motor and most of the sensory functions of the shoulder. The supraclavicular nerves, originating from the superficial cervical plexus (C3–C4), innervate the cephalad cutaneous parts of the shoulder.[6] The suprascapular nerve originates from the C5 and C6 nerve roots of the superior trunk of the brachial plexus. The superior trunk supplies most of the sensory nerve supply to the glenohumeral joint, capsule, subacromial bursa, and coracoclavicular ligament, and gives variable innervation to the skin.[11] The C5 and C6 nerve roots also give rise to the axillary nerve. Derived from the posterior cord of the brachial plexus, it supplies cutaneous innervation to the skin overlying the deltoid muscle.

Interscalene Brachial Plexus Block

The interscalene brachial plexus block (ISB) is increasing in popularity, with 42% of patients undergoing shoulder arthroplasty in the United States receiving an ISB.[50] The block is performed at the level of the sixth cervical vertebra at the C5 and C6 nerve root and superior trunk level of the brachial plexus.[7] Successful blockade achieves analgesia at the lateral two-thirds of the clavicle, the proximal humerus, and the glenohumeral joint.[6,11] The ulnar nerve (C8, T1) is typically spared with this block, limiting usefulness for distal procedures.

The ISB is the most commonly used block and is considered the gold standard regional anesthetic technique for shoulder procedures.[7,11] Multiple approaches have been described, including anterior, posterior, and lateral, with advantages and disadvantages to each.[6,11] However, substantial risks are inherent to ISB, including central and peripheral nervous system injuries, respiratory complications, and cardiovascular complications.[51] The most serious of these include central blocks with paralysis, brachial plexopathy, recurrent laryngeal nerve palsy, Horner syndrome, pneumothorax, phrenic nerve palsy, and cardiac arrhythmia. Because of the potential for serious complications, ISB should only be performed by practitioners with appropriate experience.[7] A strong correlation between complication rate and the number of blocks performed has been established.[51]

Although the use of either paresthesia or the nerve stimulation technique to locate and identify the brachial plexus anatomy has historically been used, ultrasound imaging techniques have become increasingly popular. One study demonstrated a reduced need for local anesthetic volume while achieving greater efficacy and lower complication rates, specifically Horner syndrome, with the introduction of ultrasound guidance to ISB.[52] Other studies comparing ultrasound with nerve stimulation have demonstrated an improved success rate,[53] less hemi-diaphragmatic paresis,[54] and a reduced number of needle passes to perform the block.[55] In shoulder arthroscopy, no differences were observed in block failures, patient satisfaction, or postoperative neurologic symptoms between ultrasound and nerve stimulation.[55]

ISBs may be performed as either a single injection or with a continuous catheter via a portable infusion device. A single injection provides excellent early analgesia compared with controls in the first 24 hours but has a limited duration of action.[56,57] Modalities to prolong blockade using non-neurotoxic perineural additives are being investigated. Clonidine and buprenorphine are safe as adjuvants,[6,11,58] but midazolam should not be combined with a local anesthetic.[58]

Continuous ISB with a portable infusion device adds additional complexities but provides excellent prolonged analgesia postoperatively. A single infusion catheter can be used to block the shoulder joint, and any resulting motor block is generally well tolerated.[7] Continuous ISB used in ambulatory shoulder surgery demonstrated significantly decreased pain, opioid requirements, and opioid-related side effects compared with a saline group.[9] In patients undergoing shoulder arthroplasties, continuous ISB decreased the time to discharge, had greater early passive range of motion, and decreased opioid use compared with a group receiving saline.[59]

Suprascapular Nerve Block

The shoulder joint is innervated predominantly by the suprascapular nerve and to a lesser extent the axillary and lateral pectoral nerves.[7] Using a landmark-only–based technique or in conjunction with a nerve stimulator or ultrasound device, the suprascapular nerve is readily blocked in the suprascapular fossa.[7,11,60] For more complete analgesia, blockade of the axillary nerve may supplement the effectiveness of a suprascapular block.[7,61,62]

Compared with placebo, suprascapular nerve block without an axillary nerve block effectively reduces morphine demand and consumption, nausea, and length of stay following arthroscopic shoulder surgery.[7,63] However, a suprascapular nerve block may provide inferior analgesia compared with a single-shot interscalene brachial plexus block and adds little clinical benefit when supplementing an interscalene brachial plexus block.[64,65]

A primary advantage of a suprascapular nerve block is that it theoretically eliminates the risk of phrenic nerve blockade.[11] One study demonstrated a notable effect on lung function with varying peripheral nerve blockades, and a selective suprascapular nerve catheter had the least effect on lung function.[66] Thus, potential candidates for suprascapular nerve blocks include patients with obesity or with moderate to severe respiratory disease, in whom ipsilateral phrenic nerve block and high doses of perioperative opioid would further compromise pulmonary function.[7,66] Additionally, a suprascapular block can be used as a rescue block for an unsuccessful interscalene block.[11]

Disadvantages of a suprascapular block include a requirement for 2 separate nerve block procedures when done in conjunction with an axillary nerve block. Additionally, it achieves an incomplete blockade of all nerves innervating the shoulder joint and has a limited duration of action.[7,11] It also avoids motor block to the more inferior roots of the brachial plexus (C8, T1). Risks include nerve damage, intravascular injection, pneumothorax, Horner syndrome, dyspnea, and hoarseness.[7,11,66,67]

Supraclavicular Nerve Block

Supraclavicular nerve blockade achieves a brachial plexus conduction block at the level of brachial plexus divisions, between the anterior and middle scalene at the first rib.[11] Historically of limited interest because of the risk of pneumothorax, ultrasound has reduced complications.[68–70] The incidence of pneumothorax has been reported at rates of 0.6% to 6.1%; but in a study of 510 ultrasound-guided supraclavicular nerve blocks, there was no evidence of pneumothorax.[71] Other complications of this block include vascular punctures, unintended intravascular injection, Horner syndrome, recurrent laryngeal nerve blockade, brachial plexus injury, and phrenic nerve blockade with transient hemidiaphragmatic paresis.[11,71,72] A prospective study in patients undergoing arthroscopic shoulder surgery demonstrated an excellent success rate for both interscalene and supraclavicular blocks, with less hoarseness in the postanesthesia care unit with supraclavicular blocks. There was no evidence of pneumothorax.[72]

PERIARTICULAR INJECTION

Subacromial or Intraarticular Infiltration of Local Anesthesia

Amino amide local anesthetic agents inhibit nerve signal transmission from damaged tissue by blocking voltage-dependent sodium channels within nerves and displacing calcium ions from phospholipids of the nerve membrane.[18] Injection of local agents into the subacromial or intra-articular (SAIA) space has been well described and can be performed by the surgeon at the end of a case in high volumes of 20 mL to 50 mL, with or without a long-acting catheter.[7] However, the literature has demonstrated minimal to no significant reduction of pain in most studies.[7,64,73–75]

In review of 4 studies showing a clinical benefit from continuous SAIA block with the use of a catheter, none of the studies involved open procedures.[76–79] In 4 studies showing no clinical benefit from continuous SAIA block over controls, 3 involved open procedures.[80–83] Glenohumeral chondrolysis, a devastating, irreversible complication, has been associated with intraarticular injection of local anesthetic.[84–88] Although the implications of chondrolysis may be less relevant in arthroplasty, this modality is generally no longer recommended given the limited clinical efficacy and association with chondrolysis.[7,73]

Wound Infiltration of Local Anesthesia

Liposomal bupivacaine is a long-acting local anesthetic used for wound infiltration. It uses a carrier matrix, which encapsulates and subsequently releases bupivacaine over time for sustained release of the drug.[89,90] In patients undergoing shoulder arthroplasty, a prospective randomized trial concluded that liposomal bupivacaine provided similar pain relief as an interscalene nerve block, with decreased narcotic requirements and no increase in complications or length of stay.[91] A retrospective cohort study of liposomal bupivacaine versus interscalene nerve block demonstrated lower pain scores in the liposomal bupivacaine group at 18 to 24 hours after surgery, correlating with less opioid consumption on the second and third day.[92]

Local anesthesia with classic or long-acting agents is a simple technique that may be performed during the procedure without additional expertise or personnel.[92] However, there is a relatively short duration of effectiveness and uncertainty regarding the best agent and the ideal volume of injection.[90,92] Additionally, in long-acting formulations, peak plasma levels normally occur approximately 24 hours after injection, leaving the early postoperative period relatively uncovered by the anesthetic agent.[92]

More common side effects include nausea, vomiting, and dizziness, whereas more serious yet rare complications include myocyte toxicity,

chondrotoxicity, and granulomatous inflammation.[92,93] The focus of ongoing research includes investigating the efficacy of liposomal bupivacaine in conjunction with other medication, such as intravenous dexamethasone, to decrease postoperative pain.[19] More research is needed on the cost-effectiveness of long-acting anesthetic agents[89] and its use in regional anesthesia.[90]

ORAL AND PARENTERAL MEDICATIONS
Opioids

Opioid medications act on specific opioid receptors in the central nervous system to attenuate pain-related signals.[20] They are the most effective analgesics for moderate to severe postoperative pain, but their large side effect profile must be considered.[5] Tramadol, a synthetic centrally acting opioid agonist and monoamine uptake inhibitor, has been shown to relieve moderate to severe postsurgical pain.[94] Additionally, tramadol has fewer side effects than other opioids, including no clinically relevant respiratory depression and a lower potential for abuse or dependence.[94]

One study found lower morphine consumption at 24 hours postoperatively but no statistically significant difference with regard to pain intensity, sedation, or nausea in patients treated with a combination of intravenous tramadol and morphine versus morphine alone in patients with primary total knee arthroplasty.[12] However, in patients undergoing total hip arthroplasty, one study found no significant analgesic effect with tramadol in oral doses and no difference between tramadol and placebo for any efficacy variable.[95]

Nonsteroidal Antiinflammatory Drugs

NSAIDs have opioid-sparing actions and antiinflammatory effects.[5,20,21] NSAIDs act mainly in the periphery to inhibit the initiation of pain signals by interfering with prostaglandin synthesis via blockade of the COX pathway after tissue injury.[20] COX-1 is ubiquitous throughout the body and constitutively expressed, whereas COX-2 is inducible and more specific to acute and chronic inflammatory tissues.[5,20,21] Side effects of NSAIDs include gastrointestinal bleeding, renal toxicity, and the potential for nonunion.[22,96,97]

A systematic review and meta-analysis of selective COX-2 inhibitors in total knee arthroplasty demonstrated significantly reduced postoperative pain, opioid consumption, and nausea and vomiting with no difference in blood loss during the first 24 hours postoperatively in those receiving COX-2 inhibitors.[98] Another systematic review of opioid-sparing analgesia with

COX-2 inhibitors demonstrated a reduction in opioid consumption by 35%.[99] NSAIDs are valuable as adjuvants to other analgesics for reduction in postoperative pain.[20]

Acetaminophen

Acetaminophen is widely used at moderate dosages for short periods as an analgesic and antipyretic agent.[100] The analgesic effect of acetaminophen is possibly weaker (20%–30%) than that of NSAIDs, but the drug has very few contraindications and almost no side effects at recommended doses.[34,101–103] The combination of acetaminophen with NSAIDs may enhance analgesia when compared with NSAIDs alone.[102] A meta-analysis of randomized controlled trials showed that acetaminophen combined with morphine via patient-controlled analgesia induced a significant morphine-sparing effect but did not change the incidence of morphine-related adverse effects in the postoperative period.[104]

Gabapentinoids

Gabapentinoids include the GABA analogues pregabalin and gabapentin. Both exhibit similar properties, with pregabalin demonstrating a more favorable pharmacokinetic profile with more rapid absorption and higher bioavailability than gabapentin as well as dose-dependent absorption.[22,105] Both drugs have been shown to reduce pain intensity, opioid consumption, and opioid-related adverse effects postoperatively.[22,106] The incidence of visual disturbances, dizziness, and sedation is significant with pregabalin, but the incidence of vomiting is lower.[22,105] The optimal dose and duration of gabapentinoid therapy is unknown.[106]

CRYOTHERAPY

Cryotherapy is a simple, relatively noninvasive, cost-effective adjuvant for decreasing postoperative pain.[107] Through the reduction of postoperative inflammation and swelling, cryotherapy also facilitates the oxygenation of cells.[107–112] It reduces both the metabolic rate and the oxygen demand of cells in an environment of reduced oxygen accessibility.[107,109–111] Furthermore, it can prevent neural plasticity and chronic pain by decreasing free nerve ending sensitivity, increasing nerve firing thresholds, and slowing synaptic activity.[107,108,113] However, extended periods of exposure may potentially freeze the skin.[109] Care should be taken in the anesthetized extremity, such as those recovering from a regional block.

The use of cryotherapy has been shown to reduce postoperative pain after various operations and should be complementary to other pain management strategies.[107,109,112,114] A prospective randomized study examining postoperative pain in open shoulder procedures demonstrated less pain on the first night after the operation in patients receiving cryotherapy.[115] These patients slept better on the night of surgery and reported less pain.

In a review of randomized controlled trials of pain management after outpatient anterior cruciate ligament reconstruction, 9 studies analyzed the effects of noncompressive cryotherapy.[116] Five studies reported decreased pain symptoms, whereas 4 reported no significant differences as compared with controls. Additionally, a randomized controlled trial of placing ice on a midline abdominal incision demonstrated that those randomized to receive cryotherapy for a minimum of 24 hours in time intervals determined by patient preference significantly decreased narcotic use on postoperative day one.[107]

SUMMARY

Pain control in total shoulder arthroplasty demands a broad, multidisciplinary approach with collaboration between the patients, surgeon, and anesthetist. A multimodal approach with preemptive medication, regional blockade, local anesthetics, and a combination of acetaminophen, NSAIDs, tramadol, and gabapentinoids postoperatively leads to excellent pain control and patient satisfaction.

Assessment of patients' expectations regarding postoperative pain constitutes a vital aspect of the preoperative patient evaluation. Efforts to educate and psychologically prepare patients reduces postoperative anxiety and pain. Those patients with anxiety and depression, a history of narcotic use preoperatively, and with multiple medical comorbidities are at an increased risk for less effective postoperative pain control. Minimizing narcotic use decreases opioid-related adverse effects and facilitates productive rehabilitation efforts. Ongoing research is directed at optimizing the timing and dosage of medications, using agents to prolong blockade, and fine-tuning techniques to increase efficacy and reduce complications in the delivery of cost-conscious regional anesthesia.

REFERENCES

1. Padegimas EM, Maltenfort M, Lazarus MD, et al. Future patient demand for shoulder arthroplasty

by younger patients: national projections. Clin Orthop 2015;473(6):1860–7.

2. Schoch B, Schleck C, Cofield RH, et al. Shoulder arthroplasty in patients younger than 50 years: minimum 20-year follow-up. J Shoulder Elbow Surg 2015;24(5):705–10.

3. Raiss P, Bruckner T, Rickert M, et al. Longitudinal observational study of total shoulder replacements with cement: fifteen to twenty-year follow-up. J Bone Joint Surg Am 2014;96(3):198–205.

4. Bacle G, Nové-Josserand L, Garaud P, et al. Long-term outcomes of reverse total shoulder arthroplasty: a follow-up of a previous study. J Bone Joint Surg Am 2017;99(6):454–61.

5. Jin F, Chung F. Multimodal analgesia for postoperative pain control. J Clin Anesth 2001;13(7):524–39.

6. Borgeat A, Ekatodramis G. Anaesthesia for shoulder surgery. Best Pract Res Clin Anaesthesiol 2002;16(2):211–25.

7. Fredrickson MJ, Krishnan S, Chen CY. Postoperative analgesia for shoulder surgery: a critical appraisal and review of current techniques. Anaesthesia 2010;65(6):608–24.

8. Borgeat A, Schäppi B, Biasca N, et al. Patient-controlled analgesia after major shoulder surgery: patient-controlled interscalene analgesia versus patient-controlled analgesia. Anesthesiology 1997;87(6):1343–7.

9. Ilfeld BM, Morey TE, Wright TW, et al. Continuous interscalene brachial plexus block for postoperative pain control at home: a randomized, double-blinded, placebo-controlled study. Anesth Analg 2003;96(4):1089–95 [Table of contents].

10. Wilson AT, Nicholson E, Burton L, et al. Analgesia for day-case shoulder surgery. Br J Anaesth 2004; 92(3):414–5.

11. Sripada R, Bowens C. Regional anesthesia procedures for shoulder and upper arm surgery upper extremity update–2005 to present. Int Anesthesiol Clin 2012;50(1):26–46.

12. Stiller C-O, Lundblad H, Weidenhielm L, et al. The addition of tramadol to morphine via patient-controlled analgesia does not lead to better post-operative pain relief after total knee arthroplasty. Acta Anaesthesiol Scand 2007;51(3):322–30.

13. Kehlet H, Jensen TS, Woolf CJ. Persistent postsurgical pain: risk factors and prevention. Lancet 2006;367(9522):1618–25.

14. Angst MS, Clark JD. Opioid-induced hyperalgesia: a qualitative systematic review. Anesthesiology 2006;104(3):570–87.

15. Kehlet H, Dahl JB. The value of "multimodal" or "balanced analgesia" in postoperative pain treatment. Anesth Analg 1993;77(5):1048–56.

16. Goon AK, Dines DM, Craig EV, et al. A clinical pathway for total shoulder arthroplasty-a pilot study. HSS J 2014;10(2):100–6.

17. Hebl JR, Dilger JA, Byer DE, et al. A pre-emptive multimodal pathway featuring peripheral nerve block improves perioperative outcomes after major orthopedic surgery. Reg Anesth Pain Med 2008;33(6):510–7.

18. Dahl JB, Møiniche S, Kehlet H. Wound infiltration with local anaesthetics for postoperative pain relief. Acta Anaesthesiol Scand 1994;38(1):7–14.

19. Routman HD, Israel LR, Moor MA, et al. Local injection of liposomal bupivacaine combined with intravenous dexamethasone reduces postoperative pain and hospital stay after shoulder arthroplasty. J Shoulder Elbow Surg 2017;26(4):641–7.

20. Dahl JB, Kehlet H. Non-steroidal anti-inflammatory drugs: rationale for use in severe postoperative pain. Br J Anaesth 1991;66(6):703–12.

21. Cashman JN. The mechanisms of action of NSAIDs in analgesia. Drugs 1996;52(Suppl 5):13–23.

22. Baidya DK, Agarwal A, Khanna P, et al. Pregabalin in acute and chronic pain. J Anaesthesiol Clin Pharmacol 2011;27(3):307–14.

23. Woolf CJ, Chong MS. Preemptive analgesia–treating postoperative pain by preventing the establishment of central sensitization. Anesth Analg 1993;77(2):362–79.

24. Khalili G, Janghorbani M, Saryazdi H, et al. Effect of preemptive and preventive acetaminophen on postoperative pain score: a randomized, double-blind trial of patients undergoing lower extremity surgery. J Clin Anesth 2013;25(3):188–92.

25. Dierking G, Duedahl TH, Rasmussen ML, et al. Effects of gabapentin on postoperative morphine consumption and pain after abdominal hysterectomy: a randomized, double-blind trial. Acta Anaesthesiol Scand 2004;48(3):322–7.

26. Kim JC, Choi YS, Kim KN, et al. Effective dose of peri-operative oral pregabalin as an adjunct to multimodal analgesic regimen in lumbar spinal fusion surgery. Spine 2011;36(6):428–33.

27. Straube S, Derry S, McQuay HJ, et al. Effect of preoperative cox-II-selective NSAIDs (coxibs) on postoperative outcomes: a systematic review of randomized studies. Acta Anaesthesiol Scand 2005;49(5):601–13.

28. Henn RF, Ghomrawi H, Rutledge JR, et al. Preoperative patient expectations of total shoulder arthroplasty. J Bone Joint Surg Am 2011;93(22):2110–5.

29. Mancuso CA, Altchek DW, Craig EV, et al. Patients' expectations of shoulder surgery. J Shoulder Elbow Surg 2002;11(6):541–9.

30. O'Malley KJ, Roddey TS, Gartsman GM, et al. Outcome expectancies, functional outcomes, and expectancy fulfillment for patients with shoulder problems. Med Care 2004;42(2):139–46.

31. Mondloch MV, Cole DC, Frank JW. Does how you do depend on how you think you'll do? A systematic review of the evidence for a relation between patients' recovery expectations and health outcomes. CMAJ 2001;165(2):174–9.

32. Henn RF, Kang L, Tashjian RZ, et al. Patients' preoperative expectations predict the outcome of rotator cuff repair. J Bone Joint Surg Am 2007;89(9):1913–9.

33. Mancuso CA, Graziano S, Briskie LM, et al. Randomized trials to modify patients' preoperative expectations of hip and knee arthroplasties. Clin Orthop 2008;466(2):424–31.

34. Kehlet H, Dahl JB. Anaesthesia, surgery, and challenges in postoperative recovery. Lancet 2003; 362(9399):1921–8.

35. Cho C-H, Seo H-J, Bae K-C, et al. The impact of depression and anxiety on self-assessed pain, disability, and quality of life in patients scheduled for rotator cuff repair. J Shoulder Elbow Surg 2013;22(9):1160–6.

36. Mollon B, Mahure SA, Ding DY, et al. The influence of a history of clinical depression on perioperative outcomes in elective total shoulder arthroplasty: a ten-year national analysis. Bone Joint J 2016;98-B(6):818–24.

37. Koorevaar RCT, van 't Riet E, Gerritsen MJJ, et al. The influence of preoperative and postoperative psychological symptoms on clinical outcome after shoulder surgery: a prospective longitudinal cohort study. PLoS One 2016;11(11):e0166555.

38. Roh YH, Lee BK, Noh JH, et al. Effect of depressive symptoms on perceived disability in patients with chronic shoulder pain. Arch Orthop Trauma Surg 2012;132(9):1251–7.

39. Rosenberger PH, Jokl P, Ickovics J. Psychosocial factors and surgical outcomes: an evidence-based literature review. J Am Acad Orthop Surg 2006;14(7):397–405.

40. Caudill-Slosberg MA, Schwartz LM, Woloshin S. Office visits and analgesic prescriptions for musculoskeletal pain in US: 1980 vs. 2000. Pain 2004;109(3):514–9.

41. Morris BJ, Laughlin MS, Elkousy HA, et al. Preoperative opioid use and outcomes after reverse shoulder arthroplasty. J Shoulder Elbow Surg 2015;24(1):11–6.

42. Morris BJ, Sciascia AD, Jacobs CA, et al. Preoperative opioid use associated with worse outcomes after anatomic shoulder arthroplasty. J Shoulder Elbow Surg 2016;25(4):619–23.

43. Lawrence JTR, London N, Bohlman HH, et al. Preoperative narcotic use as a predictor of clinical outcome: results following anterior cervical arthrodesis. Spine 2008;33(19):2074–8.

44. Fisher DA, Dierckman B, Watts MR, et al. Looks good but feels bad: factors that contribute to poor results after total knee arthroplasty. J Arthroplasty 2007;22(6 Suppl 2):39–42.

45. Lee D, Armaghani S, Archer KR, et al. Preoperative opioid use as a predictor of adverse postoperative self-reported outcomes in patients undergoing spine surgery. J Bone Joint Surg Am 2014;96(11):e89.

46. Morris BJ, Mir HR. The opioid epidemic: impact on orthopaedic surgery. J Am Acad Orthop Surg 2015;23(5):267–71.

47. Massey GM, Dodds HN, Roberts CS, et al. Toxicology screening in orthopedic trauma patients predicting duration of prescription opioid use. J Addict Dis 2005;24(4):31–41.

48. Morris BJ, Zumsteg JW, Archer KR, et al. Narcotic use and postoperative doctor shopping in the orthopaedic trauma population. J Bone Joint Surg Am 2014;96(15):1257–62.

49. Tashjian RZ, Henn RF, Kang L, et al. The effect of comorbidity on self-assessed function in patients with a chronic rotator cuff tear. J Bone Joint Surg Am 2004;86-A(2):355–62.

50. Gabriel RA, Nagrebetsky A, Kaye AD, et al. The patterns of utilization of interscalene nerve blocks for total shoulder arthroplasty. Anesth Analg 2016; 123(3):758–61.

51. Lenters TR, Davies J, Matsen FA. The types and severity of complications associated with interscalene brachial plexus block anesthesia: local and national evidence. J Shoulder Elbow Surg 2007; 16(4):379–87.

52. Girdler-Hardy TP, Webb C, Menon G. Improved safety and efficacy of ultrasound-guided interscalene nerve block vs a nerve-stimulator guided technique. Br J Anaesth 2015;115(3):474–5.

53. Kapral S, Greher M, Huber G, et al. Ultrasonographic guidance improves the success rate of interscalene brachial plexus blockade. Reg Anesth Pain Med 2008;33(3):253–8.

54. Ghodki PS, Singh ND. Incidence of hemidiaphragmatic paresis after peripheral nerve stimulator versus ultrasound guided interscalene brachial plexus block. J Anaesthesiol Clin Pharmacol 2016;32(2):177–81.

55. Liu SS, Zayas VM, Gordon MA, et al. A prospective, randomized, controlled trial comparing ultrasound versus nerve stimulator guidance for interscalene block for ambulatory shoulder surgery for postoperative neurological symptoms. Anesth Analg 2009;109(1):265–71.

56. Al-Kaisy A, McGuire G, Chan VW, et al. Analgesic effect of interscalene block using low-dose bupivacaine for outpatient arthroscopic

shoulder surgery. Reg Anesth Pain Med 1998; 23(5):469–73.

57. Hadzic A, Williams BA, Karaca PE, et al. For outpatient rotator cuff surgery, nerve block anesthesia provides superior same-day recovery over general anesthesia. Anesthesiology 2005;102(5):1001–7.

58. Williams BA, Hough KA, Tsui BYK, et al. Neurotoxicity of adjuvants used in perineural anesthesia and analgesia in comparison with ropivacaine. Reg Anesth Pain Med 2011;36(3):225–30.

59. Ilfeld BM, Vandenborne K, Duncan PW, et al. Ambulatory continuous interscalene nerve blocks decrease the time to discharge readiness after total shoulder arthroplasty: a randomized, triple-masked, placebo-controlled study. Anesthesiology 2006;105(5):999–1007.

60. Harmon D, Hearty C. Ultrasound-guided suprascapular nerve block technique. Pain Physician 2007;10(6):743–6.

61. Price DJ. The shoulder block: a new alternative to interscalene brachial plexus blockade for the control of postoperative shoulder pain. Anaesth Intensive Care 2007;35(4):575–81.

62. Price DJ. Axillary (circumflex) nerve block used in association with suprascapular nerve block for the control of pain following total shoulder joint replacement. Reg Anesth Pain Med 2008;33(3): 280–1.

63. Ritchie ED, Tong D, Chung F, et al. Suprascapular nerve block for postoperative pain relief in arthroscopic shoulder surgery: a new modality? Anesth Analg 1997;84(6):1306–12.

64. Singelyn FJ, Lhotel L, Fabre B. Pain relief after arthroscopic shoulder surgery: a comparison of intraarticular analgesia, suprascapular nerve block, and interscalene brachial plexus block. Anesth Analg 2004;99(2):589–92 [Table of contents].

65. Neal JM, McDonald SB, Larkin KL, et al. Suprascapular nerve block prolongs analgesia after nonarthroscopic shoulder surgery but does not improve outcome. Anesth Analg 2003;96(4): 982–6 [Table of contents].

66. Auyong DB, Yuan SC, Choi DS, et al. A double-blind randomized comparison of continuous interscalene, supraclavicular, and suprascapular blocks for total shoulder arthroplasty. Reg Anesth Pain Med 2017;42(3):302–9.

67. Dangoisse MJ, Wilson DJ, Glynn CJ. MRI and clinical study of an easy and safe technique of suprascapular nerve blockade. Acta Anaesthesiol Belg 1994;45(2):49–54.

68. Güzeldemir ME. Pneumothorax and supraclavicular block. Anesth Analg 1993;76(3):685.

69. Chan VWS, Perlas A, Rawson R, et al. Ultrasound-guided supraclavicular brachial plexus block. Anesth Analg 2003;97(5):1514–7.

70. Beach ML, Sites BD, Gallagher JD. Use of a nerve stimulator does not improve the efficacy of ultrasound-guided supraclavicular nerve blocks. J Clin Anesth 2006;18(8):580–4.

71. Perlas A, Lobo G, Lo N, et al. Ultrasound-guided supraclavicular block: outcome of 510 consecutive cases. Reg Anesth Pain Med 2009;34(2):171–6.

72. Liu SS, Gordon MA, Shaw PM, et al. A prospective clinical registry of ultrasound-guided regional anesthesia for ambulatory shoulder surgery. Anesth Analg 2010;111(3):617–23.

73. Bjørnholdt KT, Jensen JM, Bendtsen TF, et al. Local infiltration analgesia versus continuous interscalene brachial plexus block for shoulder replacement pain: a randomized clinical trial. Eur J Orthop Surg Traumatol 2015;25(8):1245–52.

74. Laurila PA, Löppönen A, Kanga-Saarela T, et al. Interscalene brachial plexus block is superior to subacromial bursa block after arthroscopic shoulder surgery. Acta Anaesthesiol Scand 2002;46(8): 1031–6.

75. Muittari PA, Nelimarkka O, Seppälä T, et al. Comparison of the analgesic effects of intrabursal oxycodone and bupivacaine after acromioplasty. J Clin Anesth 1999;11(1):11–6.

76. Barber FA, Herbert MA. The effectiveness of an anesthetic continuous-infusion device on postoperative pain control. Arthroscopy 2002;18(1):76–81.

77. Harvey GP, Chelly JE, AlSamsam T, et al. Patient-controlled ropivacaine analgesia after arthroscopic subacromial decompression. Arthroscopy 2004;20(5):451–5.

78. Savoie FH, Field LD, Jenkins RN, et al. The pain control infusion pump for postoperative pain control in shoulder surgery. Arthroscopy 2000;16(4): 339–42.

79. Axelsson K, Nordenson U, Johanzon E, et al. Patient-controlled regional analgesia (PCRA) with ropivacaine after arthroscopic subacromial decompression. Acta Anaesthesiol Scand 2003; 47(8):993–1000.

80. Coghlan JA, Forbes A, McKenzie D, et al. Efficacy of subacromial ropivacaine infusion for rotator cuff surgery. A randomized trial. J Bone Joint Surg Am 2009;91(7):1558–67.

81. Banerjee SS, Pulido P, Adelson WS, et al. The efficacy of continuous bupivacaine infiltration following arthroscopic rotator cuff repair. Arthroscopy 2008;24(4):397–402.

82. Boss AP, Maurer T, Seiler S, et al. Continuous subacromial bupivacaine infusion for postoperative analgesia after open acromioplasty and rotator cuff repair: preliminary results. J Shoulder Elbow Surg 2004;13(6):630–4.

83. Eroglu A. A comparison of patient-controlled subacromial and i.v. analgesia after open acromioplasty surgery. Br J Anaesth 2006;96(4):497–501.

84. Bailie DS, Ellenbecker TS. Severe chondrolysis after shoulder arthroscopy: a case series. J Shoulder Elbow Surg 2009;18(5):742–7.

85. Chu CR, Coyle CH, Chu CT, et al. In vivo effects of single intra-articular injection of 0.5% bupivacaine on articular cartilage. J Bone Joint Surg Am 2010; 92(3):599–608.

86. Anderson SL, Buchko JZ, Taillon MR, et al. Chondrolysis of the glenohumeral joint after infusion of bupivacaine through an intra-articular pain pump catheter: a report of 18 cases. Arthroscopy 2010; 26(4):451–61.

87. Wiater BP, Neradilek MB, Polissar NL, et al. Risk factors for chondrolysis of the glenohumeral joint: a study of three hundred and seventy-five shoulder arthroscopic procedures in the practice of an individual community surgeon. J Bone Joint Surg Am 2011;93(7):615–25.

88. Sung C-M, Hah Y-S, Kim J-S, et al. Cytotoxic effects of ropivacaine, bupivacaine, and lidocaine on rotator cuff tenofibroblasts. Am J Sports Med 2014;42(12):2888–96.

89. Chahar P, Cummings KC. Liposomal bupivacaine: a review of a new bupivacaine formulation. J Pain Res 2012;5:257–64.

90. Tong YCI, Kaye AD, Urman RD. Liposomal bupivacaine and clinical outcomes. Best Pract Res Clin Anaesthesiol 2014;28(1):15–27.

91. Okoroha KR, Lynch JR, Keller RA, et al. Liposomal bupivacaine versus interscalene nerve block for pain control after shoulder arthroplasty: a prospective randomized trial. J Shoulder Elbow Surg 2016;25(11):1742–8.

92. Hannan CV, Albrecht MJ, Petersen SA, et al. Liposomal bupivacaine vs interscalene nerve block for pain control after shoulder arthroplasty: a retrospective cohort analysis. Am J Orthop (Belle Mead NJ) 2016;45(7):424–30.

93. Lambrechts M, O'Brien MJ, Savoie FH, et al. Liposomal extended-release bupivacaine for postsurgical analgesia. Patient Prefer Adherence 2013;7: 885–90.

94. Scott LJ, Perry CM. Tramadol: a review of its use in perioperative pain. Drugs 2000;60(1):139–76.

95. Stubhaug A, Grimstad J, Breivik H. Lack of analgesic effect of 50 and 100 mg oral tramadol after orthopaedic surgery: a randomized, double-blind, placebo and standard active drug comparison. Pain 1995;62(1):111–8.

96. Glassman SD, Rose SM, Dimar JR, et al. The effect of postoperative nonsteroidal anti-inflammatory drug administration on spinal fusion. Spine 1998; 23(7):834–8.

97. Li Q, Zhang Z, Cai Z. High-dose ketorolac affects adult spinal fusion: a meta-analysis of the effect of perioperative nonsteroidal anti-inflammatory drugs on spinal fusion. Spine 2011;36(7):E461–8.

98. Lin J, Zhang L, Yang H. Perioperative administration of selective cyclooxygenase-2 inhibitors for postoperative pain management in patients after total knee arthroplasty. J Arthroplasty 2013;28(2): 207–13.e2.

99. Rømsing J, Møiniche S, Mathiesen O, et al. Reduction of opioid-related adverse events using opioid-sparing analgesia with COX-2 inhibitors lacks documentation: a systematic review. Acta Anaesthesiol Scand 2005;49(2):133–42.

100. Remy C, Marret E, Bonnet F. State of the art of paracetamol in acute pain therapy. Curr Opin Anaesthesiol 2006;19(5):562–5.

101. Rømsing J, Møiniche S, Dahl JB. Rectal and parenteral paracetamol, and paracetamol in combination with NSAIDs, for postoperative analgesia. Br J Anaesth 2002;88(2):215–26.

102. Hyllested M, Jones S, Pedersen JL, et al. Comparative effect of paracetamol, NSAIDs or their combination in postoperative pain management: a qualitative review. Br J Anaesth 2002;88(2): 199–214.

103. Viel E, Langlade A, Osman M, et al. Propacetamol: from basic action to clinical utilization. Ann Fr Anesth Reanim 1999;18(3):332–40 [in French].

104. Remy C, Marret E, Bonnet F. Effects of acetaminophen on morphine side-effects and consumption after major surgery: meta-analysis of randomized controlled trials. Br J Anaesth 2005;94(4):505–13.

105. Zhang J, Ho K-Y, Wang Y. Efficacy of pregabalin in acute postoperative pain: a meta-analysis. Br J Anaesth 2011;106(4):454–62.

106. Tiippana EM, Hamunen K, Kontinen VK, et al. Do surgical patients benefit from perioperative gabapentin/pregabalin? A systematic review of efficacy and safety. Anesth Analg 2007;104(6):1545–56 [Table of contents].

107. Watkins AA, Johnson TV, Shrewsberry AB, et al. Ice packs reduce postoperative midline incision pain and narcotic use: a randomized controlled trial. J Am Coll Surg 2014;219(3):511–7.

108. Ernst E, Fialka V. Ice freezes pain? A review of the clinical effectiveness of analgesic cold therapy. J Pain Symptom Manage 1994;9(1):56–9.

109. McDowell JH, McFarland EG, Nalli BJ. Use of cryotherapy for orthopaedic patients. Orthop Nurs 1994;13(5):21–30.

110. Muldoon J. Skin cooling, pain and chronic wound healing progression. Br J Community Nurs 2006; 11(3):S21. S24-5.

111. Nadler SF, Weingand K, Kruse RJ. The physiologic basis and clinical applications of cryotherapy and thermotherapy for the pain practitioner. Pain Physician 2004;7(3):395–9.

112. Swenson C, Swärd L, Karlsson J. Cryotherapy in sports medicine. Scand J Med Sci Sports 1996; 6(4):193–200.

113. Butterworth JF, Walker FO, Neal JM. Cooling potentiates lidocaine inhibition of median nerve sensory fibers. Anesth Analg 1990;70(5): 507–11.

114. Akan M, Misirlioğlu A, Yildirim S, et al. Ice application to minimize pain in the split-thickness skin graft donor site. Aesthetic Plast Surg 2003;27(4): 305–7.

115. Speer KP, Warren RF, Horowitz L. The efficacy of cryotherapy in the postoperative shoulder. J Shoulder Elbow Surg 1996;5(1):62–8.

116. Secrist ES, Freedman KB, Ciccotti MG, et al. Pain management after outpatient anterior cruciate ligament reconstruction: a systematic review of randomized controlled trials. Am J Sports Med 2016;44(9):2435–47.

The Role of Superior Capsule Reconstruction in Rotator Cuff Tears

Paul Sethi, MD[a],*, Wm. Grant Franco, BS[b]

KEYWORDS

- Massive rotator cuff repair • Dermal graft • Superior capsule reconstruction • Diagnosis
- Surgical technique

KEY POINTS

- Massive and irreparable rotator cuffs are a challenging problem to treat.
- Although partial repair, debridement, and muscle transfer are all viable options, there is no clear algorithm to determine treatment plan for these patients.
- Superior capsule reconstruction may be an option for a specific subset of this population.

INTRODUCTION

The treatment of massive irreparable rotator cuff tendon tears is a consistent challenge for physicians. When treating a patient with a chronic tear with a high grade of fatty degeneration,[1–6] tendon retraction,[1,2] and muscle atrophy,[1,3–6] the physician is left with only a few options because the risk of recurrent tear and persistent pain remain high.

Current nonprosthetic treatment options include debridement and subacromial decompression,[7–10] partial rotator cuff repair,[11–17] bridging rotator cuff reconstruction with a graft,[18–23] and latissimus dorsi transfer[24–29]; although each has different factors that limit their clinical application. Reverse shoulder arthroplasty is a reliable solution,[30–33] but it is not optimal for patients in their 40s and 50s. At the time of this publication, balloon interposition is not an available option in North America.

In 2007, Mihata[34] described the superior capsule reconstruction (SCR) as a method to restore superior stability and muscle balance in the shoulder joint without repairing the supraspinatus and infraspinatus tendon tears.[35–38]

This was as an alternative solution for the patient who had an irreparable rotator cuff with a low grade of glenohumeral arthritis, underscored by the inability to perform reverse shoulder arthroplasty in Japan during that same period. Since that time, Mihata has reported on more than 100 subjects. These reports, along with numerous (unreviewed) anecdotal reports, suggest significant clinical benefit.

RELEVANT ANATOMY

The glenohumeral joint is a complex structure that is the most mobile joint in the human body. The rotator cuff, deltoid, and biceps muscles are the primary dynamic stabilizers of the shoulder and are responsible for the maintenance of the force couples and keeping the humeral head centered within the glenoid during movement.[39,40]

The superior capsule is continuous with the rotator cable. The shoulder capsule comprises the anterior band of the inferior glenohumeral ligament, the inferior pouch, the posterior band of the inferior glenohumeral ligament, the middle glenohumeral ligament, the superior

No conflict (Wm.G. Franco). Royalty and consulting Arthrex (P. Sethi). No direct conflict with anything in this article.

[a] ONS Sports and Shoulder Service, ONS Foundation for Clinical Research and Education, 6 Greenwich Office Park, 40 Valley Drive, Greenwich, CT 06831, USA; [b] ONS Foundation for Clinical Research and Education, 6 Greenwich Office Park, 40 Valley Drive, Greenwich, CT 06831, USA

* Corresponding author.

E-mail address: sethi@onsmd.com

glenohumeral ligament, and the superior capsule. The superior capsule is a thin fibrous structure that spans from the greater tuberosity across the joint space to the superior portion of the glenoid.[41] The superior capsule is connected to between 30% and 61% of the greater tuberosity and can have a larger footprint on the greater tuberosity than the supraspinatus. There is some debate about how thick the tissue is that makes up the superior capsule. One study found that it was between 1.32 mm and 4.47 mm, and another found the thickness to be between 1.6 mm and 0.4 mm.[42–45] The superior capsule has a reverse trampoline effect that keeps the humeral head from contacting the acromion.[41]

The function of the shoulder superior capsule is to act as the main static stabilizer of the glenohumeral joint. A defect in the superior capsule secondary to a large rotator cuff tear results in increased glenohumeral translation in all directions.[46,47]

DIAGNOSIS AND INDICATIONS

The accurate diagnosis of an irreparable rotator cuff is made through patient history, physical examination, and MRI.

Advanced rotator cuff disease with corresponding Goutallier grade 3 and 4 changes and irreparable rotator cuff repairs that have not responded to nonoperative measures are candidates for this procedure.

Hamada 4 changes or greater, advanced arthritic changes, and poor deltoid function are all relative contraindications to this procedure.

SURGICAL TECHNIQUE

The patient is positioned in either beach chair or lateral decubitus position per surgeon preference. After appropriate positioning, padding, surgical time out, and antibiotic administration, the procedure is started.

Arthroscopic evaluation of the glenohumeral joint is completed. Loose flaps, loose bodies, chondral flaps, suture material, and debris are debrided.

Careful evaluation of the subscapularis is carried out with a posterior lever push. The subscapularis is repaired as indicated, although a low threshold for repair is maintained to help address a balanced force couple.

The biceps is tenotomized or tenodesed per surgeon preference. The authors recommend that this is done early in the procedure (if arthroscopic tenodesis is selected) because it is progressively more difficult as the case evolves.

Evaluation of the subacromial space is performed. A comprehensive bursectomy is performed. Clear delineation between rotator cuff and bursa must be made. The tendon will not extend past the lateral tuberosity; this may help to define the residual infraspinatus. Assessment of rotator cuff mobility is carried out (Fig. 1). If there is reasonable quality tissue that may be repaired in a low-tension fashion, this repair is completed, and the SCR is aborted. Superior graft augmentation with a thinner 1 mm dermal graft is considered in this setting based on the preoperative assessment of tissue. Acromioplasty is routinely performed.

The arthroscope is placed in the posteromedial portal for viewing. The medial glenoid is then prepared. The superior labrum is thinned but not entirely debrided. The superior glenoid has soft tissue removed from the coracoid and then posteriorly. Residual rotator cuff is left intact. A probe can be used to lift up and move this tissue during the glenoid preparation. This bone is then excoriated but not decorticated. Two to 3 labral suture anchors are placed on the superior glenoid. In poor quality bone, a small screw in anchor may be considered. The most anterior anchor is placed just lateral to the base of the coracoid (Fig. 2B). This anchor is placed percutaneously, just off the edge of the acromioclavicular (AC) joint. Careful attention to aim medially, away from the glenohumeral joint is critical. The second and third anchors (when there is available space for a

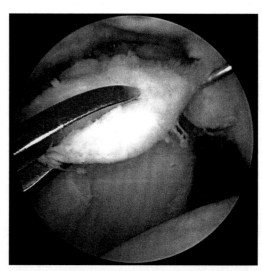

Fig. 1. Assessment of rotator cuff mobility and tissue quality. If there is reasonable quality tissue that may be repaired in a low-tension fashion, this repair is completed and the SCR is aborted.

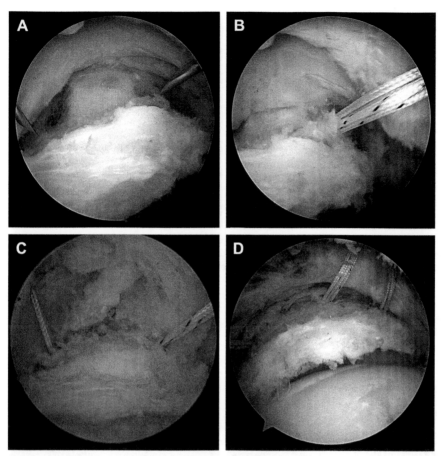

Fig. 2. (*A*) The angulation of the site where the anchors will be placed on the superior glenoid. Careful attention paid to aim medially away from the glenohumeral joint is critical. (*B*) The placement of the most anterior anchor, which should be placed just lateral to the base of the coracoid. This is placed percutaneously, just off the edge of the AC joint. (*C*, *D*) The placement of the second and third (when there is room available for a third) anchors. They are placed percutaneously inserted medial to the acromioclavicular joint, through the Neviaser portal. The most posterior anchor may be placed through a standard posterior portal.

third) are percutaneously inserted medial to the AC joint, through the Neviaser portal (see Fig. 2C,D). The most posterior anchor may be placed through a standard posterior portal. In all cases, a spinal needle is used to estimate trajectory before anchor placement (see Fig. 2A). The medial glenoid may have a variability of bone quality and, as such, anchors should be placed carefully and tested after placement.

The greater tuberosity is denuded of soft tissues and gently excoriated, not decorticated. A large cannula (ideally 12 mm) is placed in the midlateral portal. A medial row of suture anchors, loaded with tape-type sutures, are placed to facilitate a transosseous-equivalent bridge repair (Fig. 3).

Measurements are obtained between all anchors and recorded (Fig. 4). A graft is then prepared on the back table. Mihata and colleagues[35] initially described the use of a 6

to 8 mm fascia lata autograft; however, a thick (3.0 mm) dermal allograft is typically used in North America.[48] Alternate graft options are being explored. A 10 mm sleeve (or rim) of tissue is added on all 4 sides of the graft to create ideal coverage. Anatomically, the superior capsule inserts over the entire greater tuberosity, so an effort to cover the tuberosity with graft is made. Accurately placed punch holes are created in the 4 corresponding positions to match the 4 anchors that have already been placed. These holes facilitate suture sliding. Small markings are made on the lateral edges of the graft to help with orientation once the graft is delivered to the joint.

Once the appropriate graft size has been measured, if the infraspinatus is partially repairable to the tuberosity, it is done at this point. The additional sutures in the posteromedial greater tuberosity anchor may be used for

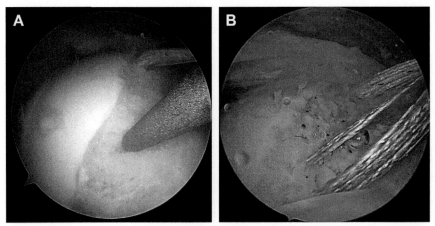

Fig. 3. (*A*, *B*) A medial row of suture anchors are placed on the humeral head. The anchors are loaded with tape-type sutures and placed through a large cannula (ideally 12 mm) in the midlateral portal. The medial row of anchors is placed to facilitate a transosseous-equivalent bridge repair.

repair. Repair before measurement may result in an undersized graft and compromised healing.

The graft is then prepared for passage. Methodical suture management is the key step component of graft passage. The graft is held up to the cannula. Each set of sutures is regrasped, passed through the graft, and brought out into a quadrant of the cannula;

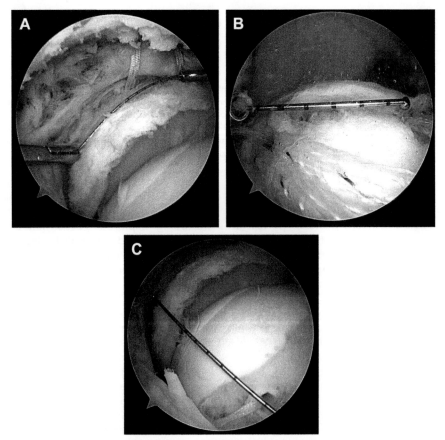

Fig. 4. Measurements between (*A*) the medial anchors, (*B*) the lateral anchors, and (*C*) the medial and lateral anchors are taken using a ruler. These measurements are used to prepare the 3 mm acellular dermal allograft.

this helps identify any unintended suture tangles. Small slits may be placed in the cannula bladder, or the sutures may be clamped to the drapes, to help this alignment (Fig. 5).

Once the sutures are all passed through the graft, and organized on the field, the graft is passed (see Fig. 5).

A combination of a push and a pull technique on the medial sutures are used to draw the graft into the joint. A gentle combination and a grasper to push the graft are used so that high stresses are not placed on the glenoid anchors (Fig. 6).

The graft is secured and tied down medially (see Fig. 6). The medial sutures may be secured in a variety of methods. Two or 3 simple knot configurations, a double pulley, or 2 (or 3) mattress sutures are all options. An additional luggage tag suture may be placed through the Neviaser portal and into the middle of the medial graft may facilitate graft passage. Each additional medial suture adds to the risk of suture confusion. The authors prefer 2 medial anchors with a double pulley technique.

The sutures in the medial row of the greater tuberosity are crossed over the graft and secured with 2 additional suture anchors laterally in a transosseous-equivalent style repair (Fig. 7). This is done with 20° to 30° of arm abduction. The graft should not be placed with laxity. The authors do not routinely link the medial row of sutures together, although this is an option.

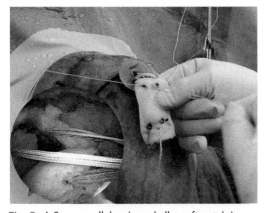

Fig. 5. A 3 mm acellular dermal allograft patch is prepared for passage. Sutures are passed through the graft outside the body using the intraarticular measurements. Methodical suture management is the key component of graft passage. Each set of sutures is regrasped and brought out into a quadrant of the cannula; this will help identify any unintended suture tangles. The sutures are clamped to the drapes to help with the alignment (small slits may be placed in the cannula bladder and may be used as well).

The weaker link on this construct is medial (not lateral), and this can add to suture confusion.

The graft is sutured to the infraspinatus with 2 to 3 sutures in a simple fashion (Fig. 8). This a not an optional step and posterior repair is biomechanically validated to recreate stability.[49] Some debate exists on repair of the anterolateral aspect of the graft to the lateral rotator interval or subscapularis. Perhaps this anterior repair may be advantageous with dermal grafts in contrast to a more rigid fascia lata graft. That said, caution is made to not overconstrain the construct with an anteromedial repair.

Patients will wear a sling for 6 weeks postoperatively. Pendulum exercise is permitted, but formal physical therapy is not done. The progressive range of motion (ROM) is used for week 6 to 12, beginning with passive stretching and active assistive ROM and active ROM as tolerated; by week 12 the patient should have achieved the latter without discomfort. Progressive strength is added from week 12 forward with a focus on shoulder flexion, deltoid strengthening, scapular strengthening, and internal and external rotation strength. No strenuous activity is allowed for 6 months postoperative.

Patients are given opiate pain medication for the early postoperative period. This is discontinued by postoperative day 5 to 10. Most patients have improvement in pain scores (from baseline) within 2 weeks, and by 3 months are comfortable and have achieved 80% of their expected pain relief. Patients are counseled to limit activity despite comfort and improved clinical function for the full 6-month period.

DISCUSSION

Biomechanically, a defect in the superior capsule of the shoulder increases glenohumeral translation in all planes.[46] The loss of this stabilizer, in conjunction with a massive rotator cuff tear, allows the deltoid to generate anterosuperior translation and shoulder dysfunction.[35] Ideally, this dysfunction may be improved with rotator cuff repair. However, in the setting of irreparable rotator cuff disease, this pathologic function is challenging to restore.

SCR theoretically improves function by recentering the humeral head and improving glenohumeral kinematics. This theory has been borne out by biomechanical studies. Mihata and colleagues[35] demonstrated that superior capsular reconstruction completely restored superior stability of a simulated irreparable cuff tear. The SCR construct's stability may prevent

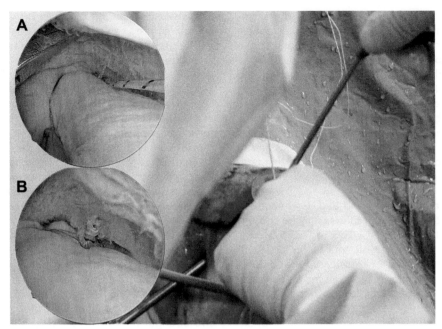

Fig. 6. A combination of push and pull techniques on the medial sutures are used to draw the graft into the joint. (A) A gentle combination and a grasper to push the graft in are used so that high stresses are not placed on the glenoid anchors. (B) The graft is secured and tied down medially.

abrasion of the graft and partially repaired tendon.[35,49,50] This restoration of stability results in a stable fulcrum, and may allow the deltoid and remaining cuff to function more effectively.

Mihata and colleagues'[36] original clinical study examined 23 subjects who underwent SCR with a fascia lata autograft. At a minimum of 2 years follow-up, the American Shoulder

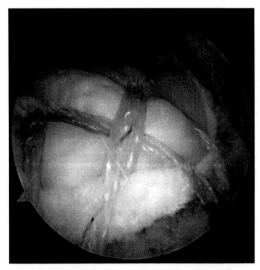

Fig. 7. Completed SCR. The lateral portion shows a completed transosseous-equivalent to a bridge style repair.

and Elbow Surgeons (ASES) score improved significantly from 23.5 preoperatively to 92.9. Postoperative MRI showed 83% of subjects had intact reconstructions with no progression of muscle atrophy.

A follow-up study confirmed Mihata's outcomes with a mean ASES score of 93.3. Ninety-two patients (92%) had neither graft tear nor re-tear of the repaired rotator cuff tendon during the follow-up period of 5 to 8 years. All subjects in this series (26%) who had played sport before their injuries returned fully to their previous sports, although most of the subjects had been playing at recreational level before their injuries.

This series also suggested that healing of the graft seems to make a clinical difference; subjects who have healed have higher ASES scores (95.5 vs 76.3) and better forward elevation.[34] They also found that pseudoparalysis was reversed in almost all subjects.[51]

Although the SCR remains a very promising option for a subset of patients with few options, some caution must be advised. Careful patient selection and meticulous surgical technique are essential. Longer term data, from multiple authors (with different graft types), are forthcoming and will require peer review. Finally, a true randomized trial comparing debridement with biceps treatment, partial repair, and SCR is warranted but it will be hard to execute and

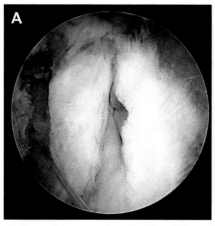 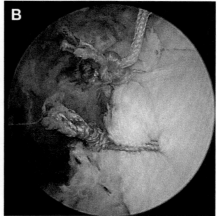

Fig. 8. (A, B) The graft is sutured to the infraspinatus with 2 to 3 sutures in a simple fashion. This is a biomechanically important step and not optional.

power appropriately given the heterogeneous nature of this problem.

SCR remains a viable surgical option, with promising early-term follow-up for a group of patients with very challenging shoulder pathologic conditions. This surgical option does not seem to compromise future revision to shoulder arthroplasty, should this become necessary.

REFERENCES

1. Bedi A, Dines J, Warren RF, et al. Massive tears of the rotator cuff. J Bone Joint Surg Am 2010;92: 1894–908.
2. Oh JH, Kim SH, Kang JY, et al. Effect of age on functional and structural outcome after rotator cuff repair. Am J Sports Med 2010;38:672–8.
3. Goutallier D, Postel JM, Bernageau J, et al. Fatty muscle degeneration in cuff ruptures. Pre- and postoperative evaluation by CT scan. Clin Orthop Relat Res 1994;(304):78–83.
4. Melis B, Wall B, Walch G. Natural history of infraspinatus fatty infiltration in rotator cuff tears. J Shoulder Elbow Surg 2010;19:757–63.
5. Melis B, Nemoz C, Walch G. Muscle fatty infiltration in rotator cuff tears: descriptive analysis of 1688 cases. Orthop Traumatol Surg Res 2009;95:319–24.
6. Oh JH, Kim SH, Choi JA, et al. Reliability of the grading system for fatty degeneration of rotator cuff muscles. Clin Orthop Relat Res 2009;468: 1558–64.
7. Burkhart SS. Arthroscopic debridement and decompression for selected rotator cuff tears. Clinical results, pathomechanics, and patient selection based on biomechanical parameters. Orthop Clin North Am 1993;24:111–23.
8. Rockwood CA Jr, Williams GR Jr, Burkhead WZ Jr. Debridement of degenerative, irreparable lesions

of the rotator cuff. J Bone Joint Surg Am 1995;77: 857–66.
9. Liem D, Lengers N, Dedy N, et al. Arthroscopic debridement of massive irreparable rotator cuff tears. Arthroscopy 2008;24:743–8.
10. Lee B, Cho N, Rhee Y. Results of arthroscopic decompression and tuberoplasty for irreparable massive rotator cuff tears. Arthroscopy 2011;27: 1341–50.
11. Kim S, Lee I, Kim S. Arthroscopic partial repair of irreparable large to massive rotator cuff tears. Arthroscopy 2012;28:761–8.
12. Yoo J, Koh K, Woo K, et al. Clinical and radiographic results of partial repairs in irreparable rotator cuff tears: Preliminary report. Arthroscopy 2010;26:E3.
13. Wellmann M, Lichtenberg S, da Silva G, et al. Results of arthroscopic partial repair of large retracted rotator cuff tears. Arthroscopy 2013;29:1275–82.
14. Holtby R, Razmjou H. A prospective outcome study of patients with large and massive rotator cuff tears: role of complete vs. partial repair. Arthroscopy 2011;27:E88–9.
15. Burkhart SS. Fluoroscopic comparison of kinematic patterns in massive rotator cuff tears. A suspension bridge model. Clin Orthop Relat Res 1992;(284): 144–52.
16. Burkhart SS, Nottage WM, Ogilvie-Harris DJ, et al. Partial repair of irreparable rotator cuff tears. Arthroscopy 1994;10:363–70.
17. Duralde XA, Bair B. Massive rotator cuff tears: the result of partial rotator cuff repair. J Shoulder Elbow Surg 2005;14:121–7.
18. Mori D, Funakoshi N, Yamashita F. Arthroscopic surgery of irreparable large or massive rotator cuff tears with low-grade fatty degeneration of the infraspinatus: patch autograft procedure versus partial repair procedure. Arthroscopy 2013;29: 1911–21.

19. Nasca RJ. The use of freeze-dried allografts in the management of global rotator cuff tears. Clin Orthop Relat Res 1988;(228):218–26.

20. Neviaser JS, Neviaser RJ, Neviaser TJ. The repair of chronic massive ruptures of the rotator cuff of the shoulder by use of a freeze-dried rotator cuff. J Bone Joint Surg Am 1978;60:681–4.

21. Heikel HV. Rupture of the rotator cuff of the shoulder. Experiences of surgical treatment. Acta Orthop Scand 1968;39:477–92.

22. Ozaki J, Fujimoto S, Masuhara K, et al. Reconstruction of chronic massive rotator cuff tears with synthetic materials. Clin Orthop Relat Res 1986;(202):173–83.

23. Post M. Rotator cuff repair with carbon filament. A preliminary report of five cases. Clin Orthop Relat Res 1985;(196):154–8.

24. Chang V, Grimberg J, Kany J, et al. Early clinical results of arthroscopic latissimus dorsi transfer for irreparable cuff tears. Arthroscopy 2012;28:E14.

25. Yamakado K. Arthroscopic assisted latissimus dorsitransfer for irreparable cuff tears. Arthroscopy 2015;31:E11–2.

26. Grimberg J, Kany J, Valenti P, et al. Arthroscopic-assisted latissimus dorsi tendon transfer for irreparable posterosuperior cuff tears. Arthroscopy 2014;31:599–607.

27. Gerber C. Latissimus dorsi transfer for the treatment of irreparable tears of the rotator cuff. Clin Orthop Relat Res 1992;(275):152–60.

28. Warner JJ, Parsons IM. Latissimus dorsi tendon transfer: A comparative analysis of primary and salvage reconstruction of massive, irreparable rotator cuff tears. J Shoulder Elbow Surg 2001;10:514–21.

29. Gerber C, Maquieira G, Espinosa N. Latissimus dorsi transfer for the treatment of irreparable rotator cuff tears. J Bone Joint Surg Am 2006;88:113–20.

30. Klein SM, Dunning P, Mulieri P, et al. Effects of acquired glenoid bone defects on surgical technique and clinical outcomes in reverse shoulder arthroplasty. J Bone Joint Surg Am 2010;92:1144–54.

31. Farshad M, Gerber C. Reverse total shoulder arthroplasty from the most to the least common complication. Int Orthop 2010;34:1075–82.

32. Simovitch RW, Zumstein MA, Lohri E, et al. Predictors of scapular notching in patients managed with the delta III reverse total shoulder replacement. J Bone Joint Surg Am 2007;89:588–600.

33. Pandey V, Willems WJ. Rotator cuff tear: a detailed update. Asia-Pacific Journal of Sports Medicine, Arthroscopy, Rehabilitation and Technology 2015;2(1):1–14.

34. Mihata T, Lee TQ, Itami Y, et al. Arthroscopic superior capsule reconstruction for irreparable rotator cuff tears: a prospective clinical study in 100 consecutive patients with 1 to 8 years of follow-up. J Shoulder Elbow Surg 2016;25(6):188–90.

35. Mihata T, McGarry MH, Pirolo JM, et al. Superior capsule reconstruction to restore superior stability in irreparable rotator cuff tears: a biomechanical cadaveric study. Am J Sports Med 2012;40(10):2248–55.

36. Mihata T, Lee TQ, Watanabe C, et al. Clinical results of arthroscopic superior capsule reconstruction for irreparable rotator cuff tears. Arthroscopy 2013;29(3):459–70.

37. Mihata T, Fukuhara T, Jun BJ, et al. Effect of shoulder abduction angle on biomechanical properties of the repaired rotator cuff tendons with 3 types of double-row technique. Am J Sports Med 2011;39(3):551–6.

38. Mihata T, Watanabe C, Fukunishi K, et al. Functional and structural outcomes of single-row versus double-row versus combined double-row and suture-bridge repair for rotator cuff tears. Am J Sports Med 2011;39(10):2091–8.

39. Mihata T, McGarry MH, Kahn T, et al. Biomechanical effects of acromioplasty on superior capsule reconstruction for irreparable supraspinatus tendon tears. Am J Sports Med 2016;44(1):191–7.

40. Terry GC, Chopp TM. Functional anatomy of the shoulder. J Athl Train 2000;35:248–55.

41. Adams CR, Demartino AM, Rego G, et al. The rotator cuff and the superior capsule: why we need both. Arthroscopy 2016;32(12):2628–37.

42. Ciccone W, Hunt T, Lieber R, et al. Multiquadrant digital analysis of shoulder capsular thickness. Arthroscopy 2000;16:457–61.

43. Itoi F, Grabowski J, Morrey B, et al. Capsular properties of the shoulder. Tohoku J Exp Med 2006;171:203–10.

44. Sheah K, Bredella MA, Warner JJ, et al. Transverse thickening along the articular surface of the rotator cuff consistent with the rotator cable: Identification with MR arthrography and relevance in rotator cuff evaluation. AJR Am J Roentgenol 2009;193:679–86.

45. Trumble T, Cornwall R, Budoff J. Core knowledge in orthopaedics: hand, elbow and shoulder. Philadelphia: Mosby Elsevier; 2006.

46. Ishihara Y, Mihata T, Tamboli M, et al. Role of the superior shoulder capsule in passive stability of the glenohumeral joint. J Shoulder Elbow Surg 2014;23:642–8.

47. Pouliart N, Somers K, Eid S, et al. Variations in the superior capsuloligamentous complex and description of a new ligament. J Shoulder Elbow Surg 2007;16:821–36.

48. Petri M, Greenspoon JA, Millett PJ. Arthroscopic superior capsule reconstruction for irreparable rotator cuff tears. Arthrosc Tech 2015;4(6):E751–6.

49. Mihata T, McGarry MH, Kahn T, et al. Biomechanical role of capsular continuity in superior capsule

reconstruction for irreparable tears of the supraspinatus tendon. Am J Sports Med 2016;44(6): 1423–30.

50. Mihata T, McGarry MH, Kahn T, et al. Biomechanical effect of thickness and tension of fascia lata graft on glenohumeral stability for superior capsule reconstruction in irreparable supraspinatus tears. Arthroscopy 2016;32(3):418–26.

51. Mihata T, Lee TQ, Hasegawa A, et al. Arthroscopic superior capsule reconstruction eliminates pseudoparalysis in patients with irreparable rotator cuff tears. Orthop J Sports Med 2017;5(3_suppl3).

Foot and Ankle

Outpatient Management of Ankle Fractures

Charles Qin, MD[a], Robert G. Dekker II, MD[b], Mia M. Helfrich, MD[b], Anish R. Kadakia, MD[c],*,[1]

KEYWORDS

• Ankle fractures • Outpatient management • ORIF • Complications • Costs

---

KEY POINTS

- Outpatient management of ankle fractures in both nonoperative and operative settings is an understudied topic that deserves greater attention given the increasing importance of cost-savings in health care.
- Although direct cost comparisons between outpatient and inpatient open reduction internal fixation (ORIF) of ankle fracture have yet to be published, the slightly lower complication profile and reduced hospital stay associated with outpatient ORIF may lead to cost-savings seen in other domains of outpatient orthopedic surgery, including total joint replacement and spine surgery.
- Further investigation into reasons for admission for ankle fractures, including fear of surgical delay, patient and surgeon convenience, and access to outpatient follow-up, is warranted to consider and improve ankle fracture management in the outpatient setting.

INCIDENCE OF ANKLE FRACTURES

Ankle fractures are a common injury in adults, comprising 10% of all fractures and more than half of all fractures of the foot and ankle seen at major trauma centers in the United States.[1] In the last decade, there has been a steady increase in the incidence as well as severity of ankle fractures, most notably in the elderly and those with osteoporosis.[2,3] Falls from standing height and sports-related injuries are the most common cause of ankle fracture.[4,5]

A significant proportion of these injuries will require open reduction and internal fixation (ORIF), a procedure not without risk.[6–9] National initiatives, such as bundled payments of care, combined with efforts to deliver cost-effective quality care, have led to interest in reducing unnecessary hospitalizations. Closer evaluation of the viability of outpatient surgery in the field of orthopedics has extended to joint replacement, cervical and lumbar spine surgery, and most recently, ankle fracture surgery. However, the epidemiology of outpatient ankle fracture ORIF is relatively unknown. A retrospective study of 476 patients undergoing ORIF for ankle fracture at a level 1 academic center in the United States identified 256 (53.8%) patients that were treated as outpatients.[10] Schepers and colleagues[3] assessed the impact of surgical delay on

---

Disclosures: In accordance with ICMJE guidelines, the authors of this study do not report any disclosures that conflict with the subject of the present study.

[a] Department of Orthopedic Surgery, University of Chicago, 5841 S Maryland Avenue Ste Mc6098, Chicago, IL 60637, USA; [b] Department of Orthopedic Surgery, Northwestern University, 240 E Huron Street # M300, Chicago, IL 60611, USA; [c] Foot and Ankle, Foot and Ankle Orthopedic Fellowship, Department of Orthopedic Surgery, Northwestern Memorial Hospital, Northwestern University, Feinberg School of Medicine, 676 North St. Clair, Suite 1350, Chicago, IL 60611, USA

[1] Present address: Attn: Kelley Shand, 259 East Erie, 13th Floor, Chicago, IL 60611.

* Corresponding author. Foot and Ankle, Foot and Ankle Orthopedic Fellowship, Department of Orthopedic Surgery, Northwestern Memorial Hospital, Northwestern University, Feinberg School of Medicine, 676 North St. Clair, Suite 1350, Chicago, IL 60611.

E-mail address: Kadak259@gmail.com

Orthop Clin N Am 49 (2018) 103–108
http://dx.doi.org/10.1016/j.ocl.2017.08.012

postoperative outcomes and found that 54 of 88 (61.4%) patients with a closed bimalleolar or tri-malleolar ankle fracture were treated on the second day following injury or later. Trends in the management of setting of ankle fracture patients who require surgery warrant additional investigation given the focus on cost-savings and quality of care in the delivery of health care.

ROLE OF NONOPERATIVE MANAGEMENT

Traditional cast immobilization is a viable option for the management of stable ankle fractures, but for those that are deemed unstable, it has been associated with poor fracture alignment and healing as well as skin breakdown.[11] Given the lack of relevant blinded prospective studies, a *Cochrane Review* comparing surgery to casting for ankle fractures was overall inconclusive.[12] In the Ankle Injury Management Trial, 620 adults with unstable ankle fractures were randomized to casting or ORIF. Casting was associated with a significantly higher rate of malunion (15% vs 3%) and a 19% radiographic loss of reduction requiring conversion to ORIF. Although no differences in quality of life, ankle motion and pain, or patient satisfaction were detected at 6 weeks and 6 months, longer follow-up is needed to determine the incidence of symptomatic posttraumatic arthritis.[11]

COST OF OUTPATIENT ORTHOPEDIC ANKLE FRACTURE CARE

Lessons on the cost-savings of the outpatient model can be learned in the field of ankle, hip, and knee arthroplasty, where the cost differential between outpatient and inpatient surgery has been reported to be as high as 30%.[13–15] However, there is a paucity of literature describing the cost of outpatient ankle fracture ORIF. Logically, early operative fixation of inpatient ankle fractures has been shown to reduce length of hospital stay, leading to significant cost-savings.[3,16,17] Interestingly, early fixation was also associated with a decrease in complications. Of note, all patients in these studies were admitted under the anecdotal concept that inpatient monitoring may lead to a decreased complication rate.[10]

Murray and colleagues[18] evaluated the costs associated with ORIF and external fixation of unstable ankle fractures in the United Kingdom. All patients were inpatients with an average cost of $4730.28 for the episode of care. The cost of care for patients with preexisting systemic disease (eg, diabetes) was significantly greater at

$5982.65 versus patients who had no medical comorbidities at $4375.00 (P<.001). It should be noted that costs in different health care models are difficult to extrapolate to that of the United States. A cost analysis of more than 58,000 patients undergoing ORIF of the ankle identified through a statewide database in the United States sought to report the costs associated with diabetic patients given the implications to value-based health care reimbursements.[19] Complicated diabetes, which was described as previous admission for ketoacidosis, systemic manifestations of the disease, or peripheral circulatory disorders, was associated with $6895 increase in total hospital charges relative to nondiabetic patients.

The cost of outpatient reconstructive surgery of the ankle and hindfoot has also been examined and offers useful information regarding cost-savings from outpatient surgery. In a recent single-surgeon series, the cost of 218 patients who underwent hindfoot osteotomy, arthrodesis, or multiple ligament repair was retrospectively evaluated.[20] A total of 20 outpatients were 1:1 matched with an inpatient cohort for demographics, American Society of Anesthesia class, anesthesia type, and procedure. Cost data were only available for 19 outpatients and 17 inpatients, and cost data regarding perioperative complications in the outpatient group, which may have been detected outside of the hospital, were unavailable, which may bias the study results. The investigators found that outpatient management reduced perioperative and intraoperative costs by 54% ($3507 vs $7573, P<.001). As expected, the largest cost difference was related to the shorter hospital stay. This difference is difficult to interpret because patients were not matched for preoperative medical comorbidities, nor did the investigators list admission criteria or reason for admission for each patient.

ACCESS TO OUTPATIENT ORTHOPEDIC CARE

Although outpatient ankle ORIF is an attractive option given the potential for cost-savings, perioperative admission is often elected to accommodate the operating room schedule, patient convenience, or other social factors, including safety of preinjury environment, social support, and access to outpatient follow-up and care. Medford-Davis and colleagues[21] used simulated patient methodology to evaluate access to outpatient orthopedic follow-up for ankle fractures discharged from the emergency department in a large metropolitan area. Simulated patient callers who were recently discharged from the emergency department with an ankle fracture were stratified by insurance status (ie, private, public, and noninsured) and tasked to call general orthopedic practices to establish follow-up. The investigators found no differences in success rate in establishing follow-up appointments between private and noninsured patients, but publicly insured patients were nearly 6 times less likely to receive a follow-up appointment for their broken ankle. Further study on access to appropriate follow-up and its impact on perioperative admission among emergency department and orthopedic providers is warranted to ensure that all patients receive appropriate treatment in a timely and cost-effective manner.

COMPLICATIONS OF OUTPATIENT OPEN REDUCTION AND INTERNAL FIXATION

As the price of health care delivery and bundled payments of care increase, there is an impetus toward minimizing unnecessary hospitalization. Greater attention has been paid to assessing the safety of outpatient surgery in various fields, including orthopedic spine and total joint arthroplasty, but there is a paucity of similar literature in the field of foot and ankle and orthopedic trauma. Evidence to support ORIF of ankle fractures in the outpatient setting is largely anecdotal.

Although the literature regarding medical and wound complications following ORIF of ankle fracture is abundant, few differentiate complication rates between ORIF performed in the inpatient versus the outpatient setting.[8] In a retrospective study of a national cohort of 4412 ankle fractures, Basques and colleagues[22] reported that the rate of adverse events to be 3.56% and readmissions to be 3.17% following ankle ORIF. The rate of surgical site infections, a feared complication after operative fixation of ankle fracture, has been described to be 6.1% for deep infection and 14% for superficial infection.[23]

In a retrospective analysis of 205 closed ankle fractures treated with ORIF, Schepers and colleagues[3] studied the impact of surgical delay on operative outcomes with a focus on wound complications. When 24 hours was used as a cutoff to distinguish delayed treatment, the rate of wound complications was 11% compared with 0% in the nondelayed group, a statistically significant finding. Similarly, when 1 week was used as a cutoff, the rate of wound complications was 13% versus 2% in the nondelayed group ($P = .023$), a finding corroborated by previous

literature.[3,16,17,24–28] Justification for postponed fixation was not included in their analysis; however, the percentage of bimalleolar and trimalleolar fractures treated early was higher than unimalleolar fractures. It may be inferred that higher energy injuries were not postponed more frequently because of soft tissue problems. When fracture-dislocations were removed from the analyses, differences in complications with a cutoff of 24 hours and 1 week remained statistically significant.

Schepers and colleagues[3] also performed a subanalysis of 101 patients with a Weber-B fracture to determine whether there was a difference in functional outcome scores at median follow-up at 43 months between the patients with and without an infectious wound complication. The median American Orthopaedic Foot Ankle Society hindfoot score and Oleurd Molander Ankle Score was 11.5 and 10 points lower, respectively, in the cohort with an infectious wound complication. The investigators emphasized the importance of early operative treatment in closed ankle fractures to achieve superior functional outcomes and patient satisfaction. Of note, the study did not specify whether patients with surgical delay were admitted before or after surgery.

Weckbach and colleagues[10] tested the hypothesis that ORIF of ankle fractures as an outpatient procedure is safe and feasible, against the anecdotal concept that inpatient monitoring for perioperative events may decrease complication rates. Collecting data over a 5-year period, the investigators found that 256 of 476 (53.8%) patients undergoing ORIF for ankle fractures were treated as outpatients. The average length of hospital stay in the inpatient group was 1.5 days. Rates of postoperative complications (9.15 vs 3.1%) and unplanned surgical revisions (3.6% vs 1.2%) were greater in the hospitalized group. These findings were statistically significant. However, the study was limited by its single-institutional sample size and inability to effectively minimize selection bias because only distribution of age and injury severity based on AO/OTA fracture classification in the outpatient and inpatient groups was statistically similar. Rates of medical comorbidities were greater in the inpatient group. The investigators concluded that outpatient ORIF for ankle fractures is a safe and feasible concept but noted that additional factors such as individual patient situation may affect the disposition of ankle fractures presenting in the emergency department.

The investigators of this review recently published a retrospective outcomes comparison of outpatient and inpatient ORIF for ankle fractures, which to the authors' knowledge is the only study to date to evaluate the safety of outpatient ORIF while eliminating selection bias.[29] Patients who underwent ORIF of closed ankle fractures were identified using the National Surgical Quality Improvement Project (NSQIP), a validated national registry previously used to study orthopedic outcomes. Patients undergoing inpatient and outpatient surgery were propensity score-matched to reduce differences in demographics, fracture type, preoperative functional status, and medical comorbidities. Medical and surgical complications, readmission, and reoperation within 30 days of the procedure were evaluated.

The authors found that outpatient surgery was associated with lower rates of urinary tract infection (0.4% vs 0.9%; P = .043), pneumonia (0.0% vs 0.5%; P = .002), venous thromboembolic events (VTEs; 0.3% vs 0.8%; P = .049), and bleeding requiring transfusion (0.1% vs 0.6%; P = .012), but when performing a Bonferroni correction for multiple comparisons, only pneumonia remained significant. They also found that although outpatient status was independently associated with reduced 30-day medical morbidity (odds ratio 0.358; 0.212–0.605), no significant differences were uncovered with respect to surgical complications, unplanned reoperations, and unplanned readmissions. Although these findings lend reassurance to surgeons who defer admission for low-risk patients, the NSQIP dataset did not specify whether admission occurred before or after surgery or both, which precluded the study from comparing truly identical groups with only a difference in surgical setting. Last, the time between surgery and initial injury could not be determined.

Despite recent evidence to support the safety of outpatient surgery for ankle fractures, access to orthopedic follow-up may be a concern, and an abundance of retrospective data exists that cautions against surgical delay.[3,21,26,28,30] Thus, further investigation through a prospective randomized approach may help fully elucidate differences in safety between inpatient and outpatient ORIF and potentially identify a safe window of timing to perform outpatient ORIF.

VENOUS THROMBOEMBOLIC EVENTS AND ROLE OF PROPHYLAXIS

Growing attention has been paid to the role of mechanical and chemical prophylaxis for VTEs given the serious morbidity associated with this complication and the potentially dissimilar perioperative surveillance associated with outpatient management compared with hospitalization. Currently, the American College of Chest Physicians recommends against thromboprophylaxis for isolated lower leg injuries because of insufficient supporting evidence and relatively low VTE incidence.[31]

In a prospective cohort of nonoperatively managed ankle fractures with no mechanical or chemical prophylaxis, Selby and colleagues[32] identified 7 of 1179 patients (0.7%) with a thromboembolic event. Lapidus and colleagues[33] performed a prospective randomized control trial of 272 patients undergoing ORIF, receiving either dalteparin or placebo for deep vein thrombosis (DVT) prophylaxis. They did not find a difference in rate of DVTs and pulmonary embolisms between treatment groups. Rates of VTE following ankle ORIF have been reported to be as low as 0.3% in the outpatient setting.[29] In addition, in a study of 4412 ankle fractures treated with ORIF, Basques and colleagues[9] reported the rate of VTE within 30 days of surgery to be 0.8%, occurring at an average of 11.5 days postoperatively. Recognition of pertinent risk factors for VTE following ankle fracture, such as history of VTE, obesity, coronary artery disease, and dependent functional status, may help identify individuals for whom thromboprophylaxis is prudent.[9]

SUMMARY

Although interest in outpatient orthopedic surgery has been fueled by provider desire to control costs within an episode of surgical care as well as development of rapid recovery protocols, outpatient management of ankle fractures is a relatively understudied topic.[34] Nonoperative management typically consists of cast or splint immobilization with a period of 4 weeks of touch or non-weight-bearing.[11] ORIF is often elected as treatment strategy for ankle fractures.[18] Although it is unknown the cost-savings that can be achieved with outpatient ORIF, outpatient foot and ankle surgery has been shown to be associated with a 54% reduction in cost.[20] With regards to surgical safety, there is no difference in the rate of complications, readmission, and nonhome discharge between outpatient and inpatient ORIF in properly selected patients with minimal to stable comorbidities.[29] Ultimately, however, the decision to perform inpatient or outpatient ankle fracture surgery should be made on a case-by-case basis by the treating surgeon. Although the incidence of VTE following ORIF is low, there may be a role for thromboprophylaxis. Currently, early recognition and treatment of VTE may decrease the rate of pulmonary embolism and mortality. Last, concern for surgical delay, patient or surgeon availability, and strength of social support as justification for inpatient admission must be examined further in order to better define the indications and limitations of outpatient ORIF as a management option for ankle fractures.

REFERENCES

1. Shibuya N, Davis ML, Jupiter DC. Epidemiology of foot and ankle fractures in the United States: an analysis of the National Trauma Data Bank (2007 to 2011). J Foot Ankle Surg 2014;53(5):606.
2. Kannus P, Palvanen M, Niemi S, et al. Increasing number and incidence of low-trauma ankle fractures in elderly people: Finnish statistics during 1970-2000 and projections for the future. Bone 2002;31(3):430.
3. Schepers T, De Vries MR, Van Lieshout EM, et al. The timing of ankle fracture surgery and the effect on infectious complications; a case series and systematic review of the literature. Int Orthop 2013; 37(3):489.
4. Daly PJ, Fitzgerald RH Jr, Melton LJ, et al. Epidemiology of ankle fractures in Rochester, Minnesota. Acta Orthop Scand 1987;58(5):539.
5. Jensen SL, Andresen BK, Mencke S, et al. Epidemiology of ankle fractures. A prospective population-based study of 212 cases in Aalborg, Denmark. Acta Orthop Scand 1998;69(1):48.
6. SooHoo NF, Krenek L, Eagan MJ, et al. Complication rates following open reduction and internal fixation of ankle fractures. J Bone Joint Surg Am 2009; 91(5):1042.
7. Miller AG, Margules A, Raikin SM. Risk factors for wound complications after ankle fracture surgery. J Bone Joint Surg Am 2012;94(22):2047.
8. Belmont PJ Jr, Davey S, Rensing N, et al. Patient-based and surgical risk factors for 30-day postoperative complications and mortality after ankle fracture fixation. J Orthop Trauma 2015;29(12): e476–82.
9. Basques BA, Miller CP, Golinvaux NS, et al. Risk factors for thromboembolic events after surgery for ankle fractures. Am J Orthop (Belle Mead NJ) 2015;44(7):E220.
10. Weckbach S, Flierl MA, Huber-Lang M, et al. Surgical treatment of ankle fractures as an outpatient procedure. A safe and resource-efficient concept? Unfallchirurg 2011;114(10):938 [in German].
11. Willett K, Keene DJ, Mistry D, et al. Close contact casting vs surgery for initial treatment of unstable

12. Donken CC, Al-Khateeb H, Verhofstad MH, et al. Surgical versus conservative interventions for treating ankle fractures in adults. Cochrane Database Syst Rev 2012;(8):CD008470.
13. Gonzalez T, Fisk E, Chiodo C, et al. Economic analysis and patient satisfaction associated with outpatient total ankle arthroplasty. Foot Ankle Int 2017; 38(5):507–13.
14. Huang A, Ryu JJ, Dervin G. Cost savings of outpatient versus standard inpatient total knee arthroplasty. Can J Surg 2017;60(1):57.
15. Aynardi M, Post Z, Ong A, et al. Outpatient surgery as a means of cost reduction in total hip arthroplasty: a case-control study. HSS J 2014;10(3):252.
16. Pietzik P, Qureshi I, Langdon J, et al. Cost benefit with early operative fixation of unstable ankle fractures. Ann R Coll Surg Engl 2006;88(4):405.
17. Manoukian D, Leivadiotou D, Williams W. Is early operative fixation of unstable ankle fractures cost effective? Comparison of the cost of early versus late surgery. Eur J Orthop Surg Traumatol 2013; 23(7):835.
18. Murray AM, McDonald SE, Archbold P, et al. Cost description of inpatient treatment for ankle fracture. Injury 2011;42(11):1226.
19. Regan DK, Manoli A 3rd, Hutzler L, et al. Impact of diabetes mellitus on surgical quality measures after ankle fracture surgery: implications for "value-based" compensation and "pay for performance". J Orthop Trauma 2015;29(12):e483.
20. Oh J, Perlas A, Lau J, et al. Functional outcome and cost-effectiveness of outpatient vs inpatient care for complex hind-foot and ankle surgery. A retrospective cohort study. J Clin Anesth 2016;35:20.
21. Medford-Davis LN, Lin F, Greenstein A, et al. "I broke my ankle": access to orthopedic follow-up care by insurance status. Acad Emerg Med 2017; 24(1):98.
22. Basques BA, Miller CP, Golinvaux NS, et al. Morbidity and readmission after open reduction and internal fixation of ankle fractures are associated with preoperative patient characteristics. Clin Orthop Relat Res 2015;473(3):1133.
23. Olsen LL, Moller AM, Brorson S, et al. The impact of lifestyle risk factors on the rate of infection after surgery for a fracture of the ankle. Bone Joint J 2017; 99-b(2):225.
24. Breederveld RS, van Straaten J, Patka P, et al. Immediate or delayed operative treatment of fractures of the ankle. Injury 1988;19(6):436.
25. Konrath G, Karges D, Watson JT, et al. Early versus delayed treatment of severe ankle fractures: a comparison of results. J Orthop Trauma 1995;9(5):377.
26. Carragee EJ, Csongradi JJ, Bleck EE. Early complications in the operative treatment of ankle

fractures. Influence of delay before operation. J Bone Joint Surg Br 1991;73(1):79.

27. Zaghloul A, Haddad B, Barksfield R, et al. Early complications of surgery in operative treatment of ankle fractures in those over 60: a review of 186 cases. Injury 2014;45(4):780.

28. James LA, Sookhan N, Subar D. Timing of operative intervention in the management of acutely fractured ankles and the cost implications. Injury 2001; 32(6):469.

29. Qin C, Dekker RG, Blough JT, et al. Safety and outcomes of inpatient compared with outpatient surgical procedures for ankle fractures. J Bone Joint Surg Am 2016;98(20):1699.

30. Carragee EJ, Csongradi JJ. Increased rates of complications in patients with severe ankle fractures following interinstitutional transfers. J Trauma 1993;35(5):767.

31. Chao J. Deep vein thrombosis in foot and ankle surgery. Orthop Clin North Am 2016;47(2):471.

32. Selby R, Geerts WH, Kreder HJ, et al. Symptomatic venous thromboembolism uncommon without thromboprophylaxis after isolated lower-limb fracture: the knee-to-ankle fracture (KAF) cohort study. J Bone Joint Surg Am 2014; 96(10):e83.

33. Lapidus LJ, Ponzer S, Elvin A, et al. Prolonged thromboprophylaxis with Dalteparin during immobilization after ankle fracture surgery: a randomized placebo-controlled, double-blind study. Acta Orthop 2007;78(4):528.

34. Meneghini RM, Ziemba-Davis M, Ishmael MK, et al. Safe selection of outpatient joint arthroplasty patients with medical risk stratification: the "outpatient arthroplasty risk assessment score". J Arthroplasty 2017;32(8):2325–31.

Current Ultrasound Application in the Foot and Ankle

Nahum Michael Beard, MD[a,b,*],
Robert Patrick Gousse, MD[b,1]

KEYWORDS

- Musculoskeletal ultrasound • Image-guided injection • Ultrasound of the foot/ankle
- Plantar fascia • Tendinosis • Tendonitis • Hydrodissection

KEY POINTS

- Ultrasound has been used in the foot and ankle for nearly 2 decades and is being used with increasing frequency and indication.
- Utilization in diagnosis demonstrates unique advantages that are complementary to other imaging modalities.
- High-resolution ultrasound is the modality of choice for needle placement, including joint injection.
- Increasing collaboration between foot and ankle surgery and skilled ultrasonographers is leading to innovation in minimally invasive treatment of common diagnoses.

INTRODUCTION

Ultrasound of the lower extremity was one of the first utilizations of Ultrasound in Musculoskeletal Medicine and continues to grow in practice and publication with diagnostic and interventional applications.[1–3] Before the 1990s, it was primarily used for the evaluation of mass and soft tissue lesions. There were early uses in joint imaging, especially with regard to characterization of the Baker cyst and in characterizing tendon abnormality.[2,3] In the last 15 years, more and more applications are being documented in the literature, further supporting the diagnostic and interventional use of ultrasound. Lower-extremity applications have been popular, likely because of the inherent strengths of ultrasound as they relate to the foot and ankle. Sufficient clarity and detail necessary for diagnosis or interventions under ultrasound are best when the structures are superficial, are discreet, and have clear landmarks; all accurate descriptors of foot and ankle anatomy. Musculoskeletal ultrasound's cost-effectiveness and absence of radiation is welcomed by providers and patients alike.[4] To date, the published literature abounds with applications of musculoskeletal ultrasound in foot and ankle diagnostics from mass lesions to nerve entrapment syndromes. Interventional applications continue to develop as well, ranging from accurate needle placement to emerging therapies for common diagnoses while also offering the foot and ankle surgeon alternative methods of performing traditional surgeries.

Disclosure Statement: Nothing to disclose.
[a] Department of Family Medicine, University of Tennessee Health Science Center, Saint Francis Family Medicine, 1301 Primacy Parkway, Memphis, TN 38119, USA; [b] Department of Orthopaedic Surgery and Biomedical Engineering, 1211 Union Avenue Suite 520, Memphis, TN 38104
[1] Present address: 1630 East Herndon Avenue, Fresno, CA 93720.
* Corresponding author. Campbell Clinic Orthopedics, 7545 Airways Boulevard, Southaven, MS 38671-5806.
E-mail address: nbeard@campbellclinic.com

PLANTAR FASCIOSIS

Plantar fasciosis is a commonly encountered condition that often requires imaging for proper diagnosis.[5] Ultrasound provides an accurate and cost-effective modality to evaluating the bands of the plantar fascia and its attachments on the calcaneus. Biomechanics of the lower extremity create tensile forces that result in disruption of the fascia, producing heel pain.[4,6] The cause of plantar fascial pain is not fully understood; however, inflammation is noted on histologic evaluation of acute disease, whereas degeneration is noted in chronic plantar fasciosis.[4] The condition is noted to affect 10% to 20% of injured athletes and 10% of the general population, with 5% to 10% going onto surgical intervention.[6,7] Sonography can be effectively used to diagnose plantar fasciosis and assess response to interventions based on a 2016 systematic review of clinical trials.[7]

On ultrasound, the plantar fascia displays the classic compact fibrillar pattern (Fig. 1). This pattern is seen when the fascicles of a ligament or tendon are visualized in the long axis and directly perpendicular to the sound beam of a high-frequency ultrasound probe. The image typically demonstrates a dense grouping of transverse hyperechoic lines with minimal spacing and close parallel arrangement.[5] When evaluating patients, multiple characteristics have been described to identify diseased tissue. Thickness greater than 4 mm, increased Doppler signal, calcific disease, and loss of both echogenicity and fibrillar pattern were correlated with painful heels.[5,8] Not only is ultrasound a preferred tool for diagnosis of plantar fasciosis, but also it has been shown to

be effective at monitoring a patient's response to treatment[8,9] Moustafa and colleagues[8] compared patients with painful plantar fasciosis against asymptomatic heels and monitored their response to dexamethasone injections. Each patient had a repeat ultrasound evaluation at their 3-week follow-up appointment to assess their plantar fascia. They noted a decrease in plantar fascia thickness and an associated reduction in symptoms, giving an objective finding to the patient's improvement during treatment. Multiple studies have found a correlation between plantar fascia thickness and pain. These changes have been described following various treatment modalities, such as nonsteroidal anti-inflammatory drug therapy, Botox type A injections, shockwave therapy, and laser therapy.[10] The use of ultrasound allows for instant and dynamic visualization of other structures in the foot that can cause heel pain. Ultrasound-guided Tinel of Baxter nerve can aid in accurate diagnosing and treatment plans. Baxter neuropathy along with medial calcaneal neuropathy can occur with or without plantar fasciopathy. Other differential diagnoses that can be visualized via ultrasound include plantar fibromatosis, foreign bodies, calcaneal stress fractures, rheumatoid nodules, plantar vein thrombosis, and rupture (Fig. 2).[4]

Measurement of the plantar fascia is an important aspect of diagnosis. In one study, men had an average thickness of 2.4 mm on the right foot and 2.5 mm on the left foot. Women had thinner fascia, with 1.8 mm bilaterally. The same study found that thickness increased with age, height, body mass index, and weight.[11] Decreases in thickness are associated with decreased pain and can be used to evaluate different treatment modalities.[10] It is

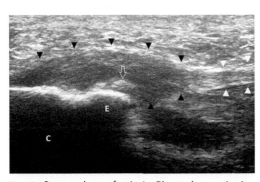

Fig. 1. Severe plantar fasciosis. Plantar long-axis view of the medial band. Normal thickness and compact fibrillar pattern is seen just distal to the origin (*white arrowheads*). The origin at the calcaneus (C) is grossly thickened with hypoechoic loss of layered architecture (*black arrowheads*) and calcific change (*white arrow*) at the enthesophyte (E).

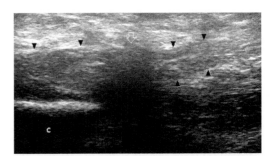

Fig. 2. Subacute high-grade partial tear of the plantar fascia. Long-axis view of the plantar fascia demonstrates complete loss of echotexture with a spheroid hypoechoic lesion (*arrow*). The surrounding fascia is edematous and thickened (*arrowheads*). C, calcaneus.

important to note that clinical context must be used in patients because one study found that every asymptomatic heel in runners had one abnormality.[9] Generally, plantar fascia thickness greater than 4 mm is considered to be abnormal but may be asymptomatic.[4,8,11]

PERIPHERAL NERVE DISORDERS

Use of ultrasound for peripheral nerve disorders is well established in the upper and lower extremities.[4,12–15] High-resolution sonography evaluation of classic abnormalities has considerable advantages over MRI with increased sensitivity (93 vs 67%) and equivalent specificity (67%) as demonstrated in a retrospective analysis of 53 patients with diverse peripheral neurologic diagnoses.[15] The common disorders of entrapment, vasculitis, trauma, neuroma, and tumor differentiation are relatively easily diagnosed by ultrasound in the context of history and physical examination.[12,15] The interactive and real-time nature of diagnostic ultrasound also offers unique advantages in the clinical decision-making process.

Peripheral nerve entrapment and mechanical neuritides are commonly treated by the foot and ankle orthopedist. These disorders can masquerade as other common causes of foot and ankle pain. Medial calcaneal, Baxters (first branch lateral plantar nerve), sural, and lateral calcaneal neuritis are in the differential of plantar fasciosis and heel pain. Saphenous neuritis can masquerade as causes of medial ankle pain, including stress fractures, osteoarthrosis, chronic deltoid sprains, and posterior tibialis dysfunction. Sural neuritis is in the differential with peroneal tendinopathy.

Ultrasound in the diagnosis of mechanical neuritides is divided into 3 distinct categories: direct imaging findings, indirect, and interactive. Direct imaging findings of nerve injury were first described in the upper extremity because of high utilization in cubital, radial, and especially the ubiquitous carpal tunnel syndrome.[12] The same principles are applied and supported by the literature in the lower extremities.[13,16] Direct imaging of the entrapped nerve is best applied at areas of nerve transition, such as exiting or transitioning between fascial planes, at muscle borders, and osseous fibrous tunnels.[12] The classic finding is hypoechoic enlargement proximal to the area of entrapment with a return to normal size or flattening or disappearance of the nerve.[12] Acute, nonphysiologic angle changes in the path of the nerve or "kinking" are also suggestive of entrapment (**Fig. 3**). As

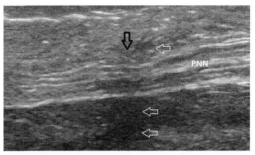

Fig. 3. Postoperative nerve entrapment at the tarsal tunnel. Long-axis view of the medial and lateral plantar nerves (PNN) with clear "kinking" of the nerves (*black arrow*) because of hypoechoic scar tissue (*white arrows*).

nerve entrapment worsens, findings will progress from subtle loss of internal echotexture to global hypoechogenicity and finally frank enlargement.[12] Cross-sectional area of a nerve has proven the most reproducible of standardized evaluations to date.[16] Ultrasound of the tibial nerve at the tarsal tunnel is very specific.[16] It revealed pathologic nerve enlargement in 100% of cases where previous electromyography and nerve conduction velocity (EMG-NCV) showed objective injury. A primary structural or compressive cause was identified in 60% of patients in the same series.[16] Recent studies of the carpal tunnel have demonstrated high specificity of Doppler signal within the nerve to clinical and EMG-NCV findings and should be looked for as suggestive in any nerve of analogous size to the median, where Doppler signal is potentially obtainable until further studies arise.

Direct visualization of nerve-specific abnormalities other than the mechanical neuritides is important to mention. Neuroma, nerve sheath tumors including schwannoma, neurilemmoma, and neurofibroma are easily visualized in the foot and ankle.[12,13,15,17] Morton neuroma is visualized as a round or oblong hypoechoic mass on average around 6 mm, with half being well-demarcated and the other half with poor demarcations.[13,18] They may appear biconcave in shape, having the appearance of a "ginkgo leaf."[18] The unique appearance on ultrasound can help distinguish Morton neuroma from other interdigital soft tissue masses such as epidermoid tumors or ganglion cyst.[18] Lesions measuring greater than 20 mm in size are likely not a Morton neuroma.[18] Dynamic visualization of the plantar surface with a sonographic Mulder click can help clarify the diagnosis[13,18] (**Fig. 4**). Nerve trauma is seen as acute enlargement

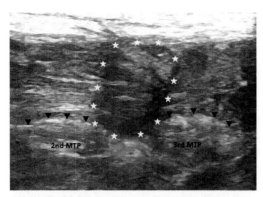

Fig. 4. Short-axis plantar view of the second web-space. A large Morton neuroma (*stars*) is seen extruded between the bright plantar capsules (*arrowheads*) of the second and third MTP joints.

with loss of internal echotexture plus or minus intraneural hematoma or frank interruption.[13] Ultrasound has a distinct advantage in the small cutaneous neuromata. The miniscule size of a distal or near terminal branch neuroma, in the range of millimeters, can be visualized under high-frequency ultrasound. Confirmation of symptoms through interventional means can facilitate a more definite diagnosis, that can allow for expedient intervention with injection or radiofrequency.[12,19]

Indirect findings include the presence or absence of other abnormality that may impinge or irritate the nerve. Nowhere in the foot and ankle is this more useful than in the tarsal tunnel, where the juxtaposition of the tibial nerve to joint, tendon, and vasculature is so intimate and the causes so diverse. Ultrasound gives excellent visualization of the tarsal tunnel contents and is comparable to MRI, and for small or subtle lesions may have an advantage over MRI.[20,21] Common ultrasound positive causes of tarsal tunnel syndrome include ganglia, talocalcaneal coalitions, varicosities, tenosynovitis, and posttraumatic/postoperative scar tissue (see **Fig. 3**).[12,20–23] Another important indirect finding that is helpful especially in the context of real-time ultrasound scanning is the evaluation of terminal innervation musculature. Denervation changes of decreased mass and change in echotexture including terminal fatty infiltration are readily appreciable.[12]

Interactive information is unique to ultrasound as an imaging modality because of real-time visualization of tissues while applying elements of physical examination or invasive interventions. Ultrasound-guided palpation to localize symptoms to visualized tissues and abnormality is helpful across all diagnostic

utilization. Needle and fluid flow interactions during injection or needle-based procedures can reveal the presence of adhesions or tethering subtle scar tissue either from direct response to the physical contact or through relative change in echotexture from the injection of fluids. Often tissue that is indistinct becomes readily visualized with fluid acting as "contrast" between it and surrounding tissues. Unique to the nerve is the ultrasonographic "Tinel." This sign is produced by mechanical stimulation of the nerve (eg, tapping) with the ultrasound probe or manually under direct ultrasound visualization. It is usually present at the area or areas of abnormality and correlates with direct nerve changes such as enlargement.[12]

Selective low-volume anesthetic injection of a specific nerve under ultrasound guidance may be beneficial diagnostically as well, especially in distinguishing causes of pain. A prime example would be a block of Baxter nerve at the level of the abductor hallucis to distinguish this common neurogenic pain in the heel from plantar fasciosis or other causes. Fluid flow during a diagnostic or therapeutic injection along or surrounding a nerve or its fascial plane may become interrupted at the site of subtle entrapment or manifest a "pop" phenomenon as flow pressure builds and then releases as fascial tethers are cleared. The combination of these interventional findings especially in the context of direct or indirect evidence of abnormality can work with the rest of a clinical examination and appropriate nerve testing to help establish abnormality and a rationale for a treatment plan.

TENDINOPATHY

The tendons of the foot and ankle are well visualized under high-frequency ultrasound techniques because of the superficial nature and dynamic access to various positions of the foot and ankle. The main limitation continues to be user dependence with likely differences between minimally trained and highly experienced providers,[24] which is yet uncharacterized in the literature. Despite challenges of user dependence, series have shown good correlation between surgical findings and ultrasound as well as MRI and ultrasound.[24–26] Tendons are visualized routinely in the short and long axis with attention to tendon morphology, size, and relationship with associated structures, especially nerves, bursae, fat pad, and bone. Doppler imaging of associated neovasculature has a role in quantifying tendinopathy that is not clearly elucidated.[25] Finally, dynamic imaging can be very helpful and is a quality unique to ultrasound especially as regards tendon disruption or subluxation. The classic ultrasound description of tendon and ligament in the long axis is the compact fibrillar pattern, which is a linear appearance of tendon fascicles that can be interrupted or lost in the form of hypoechogenic changes, discontinuity, calcification, or disorganized appearance. The short axis often in combination with dynamic images is best at revealing split tearing and other longitudinal abnormalities (Figs. 5 and 6).

The role of ultrasound has been best described in the Achilles tendon (Figs. 7 and 8) with the highest-quality accompanying studies. It is very good, 96% accuracy, at diagnosing complete Achilles ruptures and 75% accuracy in diagnosing partial ruptures compared with surgical correlation. The authors of this retrospective chart review admit these results may underrepresent the accuracy of ultrasound, however, because the examinations were performed by general radiologists with limited exposure to musculoskeletal ultrasound.[24] In less severe abnormality as in the tendinosis/tendonopathy spectrum, the accuracy is much more variable but is reported as comparable to MRI in clinical disease with sensitivity/specificity 80/49 and 95/50, respectively.[24,25] Ultrasound utilization in prognosis is still relatively poor for mild clinical disease but excellent in Achilles rupture and can be used for treatment planning.[27,28] Westin and

colleagues[28] compared operative versus nonoperative treatments of Achilles rupture and reported a high rerupture rate with 10 mm or more diastasis in the nonsurgical group measured by ultrasound at injury. There were no observed reruptures in nonoperative cases with less than 10-mm diastasis. Significantly better patient-reported outcomes using the Achilles Tendon Total Rupture Score and heel-rise height at 12 months were shown with diastasis less than 5 mm.[28] Preoperative ultrasound of the Achilles allows for accurate site marking of the rupture as well as the proximal and distal stumps and may facilitate minimally invasive repair techniques. Agreement on a standardized ankle joint angle between ultrasonographer and surgeon is advisable. Reported has been 30° of equinus, but there is no current standard.

The other tendons of the foot and ankle are easily visualized on dynamic high-frequency ultrasound. Although head-to-head comparisons with MRI have not been done, ultrasound with its dynamic or interactive imaging is extremely effective in the imaging of the peroneals and is a good early test of abnormality, including peroneal dislocation, intrasheath subluxation, split tearing, tenosynovitis, os peroneum fracture, and acute strain (see Figs. 5 and 6). All of these have distinct ultrasonographic appearances and are arguably reliable to guide treatment. Recourse to MRI or computed tomography is necessary only in cases of associated significant bony disease or for purposes of preoperative planning.[26,29–31] The abnormality of the anterior and posterior tibialis tendons is also well documented with appropriate MRI correlation with equivalent usage for these disorders.[21,32–34] Cartilaginous accessory navicular, which may be difficult to visualize on MR, is fairly easily visualized on ultrasound. Ultrasound of the other foot extrinsics and intrinsics can be quite helpful, especially at the ankle and dorsum of the foot. On the plantar surface, ultrasound can lose resolution because of the depth of penetration and sonographic densities of the plantar tissues, making MRI the preferred imaging technique with notable exception at the plantar fascia. Ultrasound continues to have excellent indications for image-guided intervention throughout.[21]

LIGAMENTOUS EXAMINATION

Diagnostic evaluation of the ligamentous structures about the foot and ankle is well described and is part of standardized training programs in

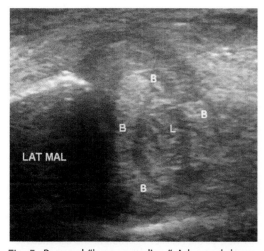

Fig. 5. Peroneal "banana peeling." Advanced degeneration of the peroneus brevis with longitudinal bundles (B) wrapping circumferentially around the oblong normal longus (L) at the level of the lateral malleolus (Lat Mal).

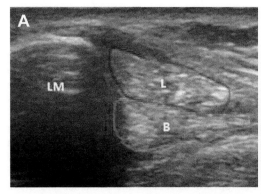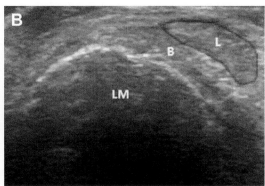

Fig. 6. Peroneal intrasheath subluxation. (*A*) Peroneus longus (L) and brevis (B) (highlighted for contrast) resting in a shallow fibular groove of the lateral malleolus (LM) with the ankle in neutral position. (*B*) Ankle in active dorsiflexion eversion. The peroneus brevis subluxes under the longus with palpable snap and pain in dynamic imaging.

musculoskeletal ultrasound. Evidence of acute sprain is characterized by disruption of the compact fibrillar pattern of the ligament edema or adjacent hematoma.[21] Chronic sprain can show loss of robust compact fibrillar pattern, and when severe, complete disorganization of the ligamentous tissue and nonvisualization.[21] Dynamic examination for ankle instability has been described but should have appropriate clinical relevance.[35] Small avulsion fractures associated with ankle and lateral column sprains are quite common, and ultrasound can be used to identify these early (**Fig. 9**). Early diagnosis is especially helpful in the case of intraarticular fractures, which can result in painful nonunion or persistent synovitis and may require more aggressive initial immobilization. In the pediatric population, such small avulsion invisible on plain films can be a marker of ankle instability.[21,36]

INJECTION

Perhaps the most common utilization in the foot and ankle is for simple injection guidance. Ultrasound-guided injections in the foot and ankle specifically have been shown to be accurate in both large and small joint and tendon sheaths (**Fig. 10**).[37,38] It also allows sufficient visualization so as to avoid intervening structures. Ultrasound is distinctly more accurate than landmark guidance for small joints and may have advantages in larger (tibiotalar, subtalar) joints if the anatomy is significantly deranged.[38,39] Increased short-term benefit of directed injections of corticosteroid in other major joints (shoulder, knee) has been demonstrated but is not yet proven for the foot and ankle.[40] Perhaps the best benefit of real-time sonographic intervention is the concept of

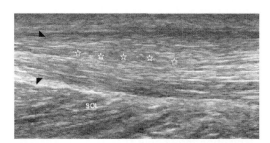

Fig. 7. Midsubstance Achilles tendinosis. Long-axis visualization reveals normal compact fibrillar pattern and thickness on the proximal end (*arrowheads*) giving way to fusiform thickening of the tendon and mild "ground glass" echotexture that appears centrally (*stars*). The distal soleus is visualized deep to the symptomatic area (SOL).

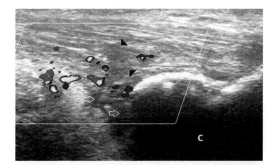

Fig. 8. Severe insertional Achilles tendinosis. A long-axis view of the Achilles insertion at the calcaneus (C) with loss of compact fibrillar pattern, peritendinous and intratendinous Doppler signal, hypoechoic regions (*arrowheads*), and irregular gross thickening of the retrocalcaneal bursa at its junction with Kager fat pad (*arrows*).

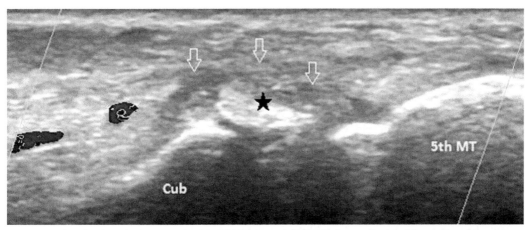

Fig. 9. Occult cuboid avulsion in an 18-year-old collegiate volleyball player after inversion injury with persistent lateral foot pain despite protected weight-bearing. Long-axis view of the lateral tarsometatarsal joint is visualized and corresponds to maximal tenderness. An intra-articular avulsion from the cuboid is seen (*star*). The joint capsule is thickened and distended (*arrows*) with Doppler signal approaching the area, consistent with secondary synovitis. Cub, cuboid; 5th MT, fifth metatarsal.

selective blockade. Selective local anesthetic application in painful joints or tendon sheaths/bursae allowing for examination or trial of ambulation while under anesthesia is well established and may correlate to surgical outcome.[41,42] Selective block is more specific than radiology findings of degeneration for determining source of pain and can result in improved success in joint arthrodesis for painful joints of the foot and ankle.[29,41,42] Selective block may not be as relevant in isolated tibiotalar joint arthrodesis for posttraumatic arthrosis in the context of long-term outcomes.[43] Advantages of ultrasound over traditional fluoroscopy for this indication include expedience in office application, allowing increased sonographer, patient, and foot and ankle surgeon dialogue.

GANGLION ASPIRATION

Ganglion cysts are filled with mucin and can produce pain due to compression of surrounding structures.[44] Because of this, they appear to contain hypoechoic homogenous fluid on examination.[45] Ultrasound aspiration and injection of ganglion cysts have become a popular treatment due to the minimally invasive execution and constitute one of the first utilizations of ultrasound guidance. Ultrasound allows for visualization of the structure's depth, dimensions, and

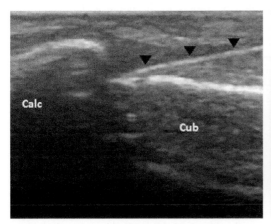

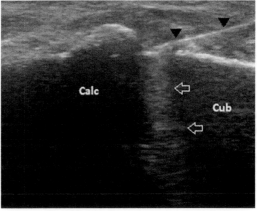

Fig. 10. Small joint corticosteroid injection. The calcaneous (Calc)/cuboid (Cub) joint is visualized in the long axis. A 25-gauge needle (*arrowheads*) is placed bevel down into the joint, and the steroid particulate is seen to flow into the joint with motion artifact (*arrows*).

proximity to nerves and vessels.[44] Thus, safe visualization of the needle entering the substance and dynamic emptying of the cyst can be noted in real time.[45] Ju and colleagues[44] found that 77% of their patients who underwent ultrasound-guided aspiration for a symptomatic lower-extremity ganglion cyst reported resolution of symptoms at 1-year follow-up. Percutaneous aspiration has less morbidity than open excision and allows physicians to conduct an ultrasonographic evaluation of a painful lesion.

SOFT TISSUE INJECTION

Needle localization for soft tissue injection independent of a joint or ganglion is well established and was first described nearly 2 decades ago.[46] As such, multiple substances have been introduced into the structures of the lower extremity with varying success,[47,48] including corticosteroid,[49] dextrose,[50] biologics like platelet-rich plasma and stem cells,[51] and even electricity.[52] Botulinum toxin has shown success for plantar fasciosis and for chronic exertional compartment syndrome.[53,54] Needle placement, without injection, used instead for fenestration under ultrasound has recently been described as a treatment of chronic compartment syndrome in a case report.[55] Independent of specific substances, ultrasound allows unparalleled real-time control for needle placement in routine or experimental models.

MORTON NEUROMA

Special attention deserves to be paid to ultrasound-guided injection of Morton neuroma. Ultrasound allows not just appropriate diagnosis but also ease of access for preferred nonsurgical treatments. A systematic review comparing the 2 methods found that ultrasound-guided injections provided better short-term and long-term relief.[56] According to a review done by Morgan and colleagues,[56] guided injections reduced pain by 66% in comparison to the 50% reduction noted in nonguided procedures. Ultimately, ultrasound provides accurate medication delivery, improved outcomes, and reduction in the amount of repeat injections given to patient and decreases the need for surgical intervention.[56]

The benefit of ultrasound lies in its cost-effectiveness and its application to multiple treatment modalities. Chuter and colleagues[57] described a series using ultrasound-guided radiofrequency ablation of Morton neuroma and found that it reduced symptoms and reduced the need for surgical excision by 85%, allowing for an in-office, percutaneous alternative to surgical treatment of these lesions.

EMERGING THERAPIES

The ability to accurately identify structures and disease as well as accurately place needles has begun to spawn innovations in treatment based around the concept of real-time interactions with the underlying abnormality. The movement from sporadic islands of clinical practice to an emergence in the literature has been slow but with increasing frequency. Treatments range from needle-based interventions and augmentation of traditional surgery with preoperative or intraoperative imaging to the development of new technologies to allow novel minimally invasive techniques.

HYDRODISSECTION

Sonographic hydrodissection is defined by the use of a fluid medium, usually local anesthetic or saline, to dissect between structures or fascial planes as directed by injection under continuous ultrasound visualization. To date, published studies and case reports are few but with increasing number in recent years. Most attention has been directed at the upper extremity with the technique used as an alternate effective means of treating carpal tunnel syndrome.[58,59] The basic technique includes identifying the region of nerve entrapment or compression and successful decompression using hydrodissection technique either in the long axis of the nerve or in the short axis, where circumferential dissection can be accomplished. The technique uses tissue treatment without direct needle impingement or trauma to the nerve and with minimal trauma to the tissues, even using needles as small as 25 gauge. Successful treatment of sural nerve entrapment has been documented in the foot and ankle.[60]

Ultrasound visualization combined with hydrodissection has been used in the case of foreign body removal, intraoperatively allowing the surgeon to insulate the foreign body from the surrounding structures with a bubble of fluid to allow surgical access.[61] When combined with accurate sonographic surgical guidance, this can minimize surrounding tissue injury during removal.[61–64] Hydrodissection can be applied in other soft tissue disorders, including tendinopathy (Figs. 11 and 12). Literature is limited to Achilles midsubstance disease. Symptomatic treatment of midsubstance Achilles tendinosis

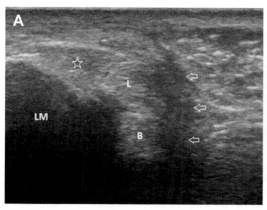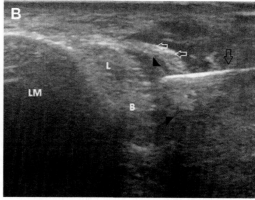

Fig. 11. (*A, B*) Hydrodissection of peroneals. A 40-year-old man after remote peroneal synovectomy with pain over the peroneals and loss of subtalar motion on his right side. Immediately after the procedure, pain decreased and range of motion markedly improved. (*A*) Peroneus longus (L) and brevis (B) at the lateral malleolus (LM). The superficial retinaculum is visualized (*star*) as is a mass of typical-appearing postoperative scar (*white arrows*) adhering to the peroneals and preventing physiologic motion. (*B*) Dilute local anesthetic is introduced under gentle pressure (*arrowheads*) by a 25-gauge needle (*black arrow*) dissecting the peroneals away from the scar, which now appear bright when contrasted with the fluid.

with hydrodissection-based stripping of the anterior paratenon away from Kager fat pad with high-volume fluid injection has been found to be effective in 2 trials to date.[65,66] This concept of treating the paratenon-fat pad junction in midsubstance disease has been recently combined with traditional percutaneous tendon stripping into an ultrasound-guided mini-open stripping/tenolysis by Alfredson[67] with good results in his series as well.

ULTRASONOGRAPHIC AUGMENTATION OF SURGERY

Ultrasound has the potential to augment many aspects of traditional foot and ankle surgery. Perhaps most helpful is the ability to use ultrasound preoperatively or intraoperatively to identify soft tissue and bony structures over and above traditional palpation or landmark-guided techniques. Assistance in endoscopy is documented not just in helping with port placement but also with offering another means of visualization. Published cases and series include arthroscopy of the hallux and several techniques at the plantar fascia.[68–70] Ultrasound guidance in

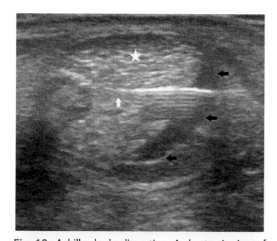

Fig. 12. Achilles hydrodissection. A short-axis view of the area of maximal tenderness of the midsubstance of the Achilles (*star*). A 25-gauge needle injects local anesthetic with partial dissection of Kager fat pad (*black arrows*) away from the lateral tendon. The needle tip (*white arrow*) is advanced directly under the tendon to facilitate further dissection.

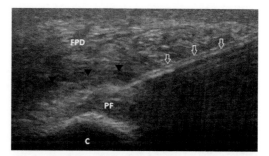

Fig. 13. Ultrasonographic fasciotomy. Long-axis view of the plantar fascia (PF) is partially obscured by a hypersonic surgical probe (*arrows*). It is debriding the proximal portion of the origin. Iatrogenic fluid is seen in the subcalcaneal bursa (*arrowheads*) separating the origin from the plantar fat pad (FPD). C, calcaneus.

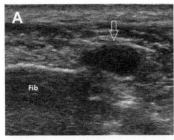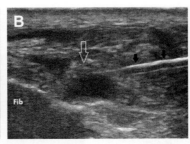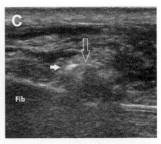

Fig. 14. (A–C) Percutaneous ablation of stump neuroma. A 75-year-old after right below knee amputation with a 5-mm fibular nerve stump neuroma. Surgical progression from left to right. The neuroma (*large white arrow*) is localized in the short axis adjacent to the fibular neck (Fib) in each image. (A) Large hypoechoic neuroma before instrumentation (*arrows*). (B) Canalization by an 18-gauge needle (*black arrows*) to the neuroma to allow radiofrequency ablation with 3-mm small joint arthroscopy RF probe. (C) After ablation. The hypoechoic structure is replaced with edema and vapor (*filled white arrow*).

open/mini-open Achilles surgery has been mentioned above with regard to the Achilles tenolysis and to foreign body removal. The arthroscope or open visualization has been abandoned by an increasing number of clinicians in favor of direct ultrasound visualization of the surgical instrumentation wielded percutaneously. New technologies include the adaptation of ultrasonic phacoemulsification technology to perform tenotomy or fasciotomy, but evidence of benefit is only at the case report level in the foot and ankle (**Fig. 13**).[71,72]

Percutaneous radiofrequency lesioning of the plantar fascia is demonstrating consistent results with mounting evidence and has been described using both needle-based and bipolar surgical devices.[52,73–77] Ultrasound has been introduced to facilitate needle/probe placement especially in the context of obesity.[52] The desire to minimize surgical trauma while maintaining transcutaneous visualization by ultrasound has led to the adaptation of traditional instrumentation in nontraditional techniques. A hook knife has been adapted in a new ultrasound-directed technique of performing a Strayer procedure.[78] A meniscotome has been used successfully to perform lower-limb decompression fasciotomies.[79] Basic technique for adapting small joint arthroscopy tools like shavers and bone burs is described and has recently been successfully used to perform a novel percutaneous osteotomy in a case of calcaneal enthesophyte fracture nonunion.[80,81] Augmentation of traditional surgery techniques and tools, although promising, is not yet well established and requires a team of highly skilled interventional ultrasonographers and orthopedic surgeons to effectively apply (**Figs. 13–15**).

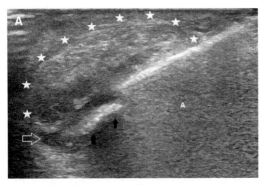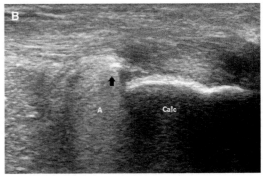

Fig. 15. (A, B) Retrocalcaneal bursectomy in insertional Achilles disease. (A) Short-axis view of the Achilles (*stars*). A 3.5-mm arthroscopic shaver is introduced via a lateral portal to debride the undersurface of the Achilles. The active shaver tip (*black arrows*) is advanced to the medial, proximal-most aspect of the hypoechoic bursa (*white arrow*) on the undersurface of the tendon. (B) Long-axis view. The active shaver tip (*black arrow*) is seen beneath the Achilles proximal to the calcaneus (Calc). In both images, portions of Kager fat pad are obscured by an active vibration artifact (A) as the shaver is activated.

SUMMARY

From its earliest applications, the development of musculoskeletal ultrasound has included indications in the foot and ankle. Inherent in the foot and ankle are attributes that make ultrasound ideal, especially the relatively superficial anatomy. As a diagnostic modality, it is relatively inexpensive, complementary with MRI, and allows for interactive diagnostics in subtle or complicated cases. User dependence and the need for highly trained sonographers continue to be major drawbacks. Foot and ankle ultrasound has been established as an effective and preferred modality for needle placement, but has in recent years moved beyond simple injections, inspiring innovation in technique and technology in treating the challenging diagnoses of the foot and ankle. Ultrasound will continue to adapt to service the foot and ankle surgeon even as foot and ankle surgery continues to guide and direct its safe and effective innovation. Perhaps this is ultrasound's greatest strength in that it can by its interactive nature draw the ultrasonographer, the surgeon, and the patient into a dialogue that facilitates care.

REFERENCES

1. Murray RO. Orthopaedic radiology: an expanding discipline. J R Soc Med 1980;73(5):320–3.
2. Meire GB, Lindsay DJ, Swinson DR, et al. Comparison of ultrasound and positive contrast arthrography in the diagnosis of popliteal and calf swellings. Ann Rheum Dis 1974;33(3):221–4.
3. Reinherz RP, Zawada SJ, Sheldon DP. Recognizing unusual tendon pathology at the ankle. J Foot Surg 1986;25(4):278–83.
4. Hoffman DF, Grothe HL, Bianchi S. Sonographic evaluation of hindfoot disorders. J Ultrasound 2014;17(2):141–50.
5. Draghi F, Gitto S, Bortolotto C, et al. Imaging of plantar fascia disorders: findings on plain radiography, ultrasound and magnetic resonance imaging. Insights Imaging 2017;8(1):69–78.
6. Wearing SC, Smeathers JE, Urry SR, et al. The pathomechanics of plantar fasciitis. Sports Med 2006; 36(7):585–611.
7. Radwan A, Wyland M, Applequist L, et al. Ultrasonography, an effective tool in diagnosing plantar fasciitis: a systematic review of diagnostic trials. Int J Sports Phys Ther 2016;11(5):663–71.
8. Moustafa AM, Hassanein E, Foti C. Objective assessment of corticosteroid effect in plantar fasciitis: additional utility of ultrasound. Muscles Ligaments Tendons J 2015;5(4):289–96.
9. Hall MM, Finnoff JT, Sayeed YA, et al. Sonographic evaluation of the plantar heel in asymptomatic endurance runners. J Ultrasound Med 2015;34(10): 1861–71.
10. Mahowald S, Legge BS, Grady JF. The correlation between plantar fascia thickness and symptoms of plantar fasciitis. J Am Podiatr Med Assoc 2011; 101(5):385–9.
11. Abul K, Ozer D, Sakizlioglu SS, et al. Detection of normal plantar fascia thickness in adults via the ultrasonographic method. J Am Podiatr Med Assoc 2015;105(1):8–13.
12. Jacobson JA, Wilson TJ, Yang LJ. Sonography of common peripheral nerve disorders with clinical correlation. J Ultrasound Med 2016;35(4):683–93.
13. Yablon CM, Hammer MR, Morag Y, et al. US of the peripheral nerves of the lower extremity: a landmark approach. Radiographics 2016;36(2): 464–78.
14. Nwawka OK, Miller TT. Ultrasound-guided peripheral nerve injection techniques. AJR Am J Roentgenol 2016;207(3):507–16.
15. Zaidman CM, Seelig MJ, Baker JC, et al. Detection of peripheral nerve pathology: comparison of ultrasound and MRI. Neurology 2013;80(18):1634–40.
16. Samarawickrama D, Therimadasamy AK, Chan YC, et al. Nerve ultrasound in electrophysiologically verified tarsal tunnel syndrome. Muscle Nerve 2016;53(6):906–12.
17. Kwok KB, Lui TH, Lo WN. Neurilemmoma of the first branch of the lateral plantar nerve causing tarsal tunnel syndrome. Foot Ankle Spec 2009; 2(6):287–90.
18. Park HJ, Kim SS, Rho MH, et al. Sonographic appearances of Morton's neuroma: differences from other interdigital soft tissue masses. Ultrasound Med Biol 2011;37(8):1204–9.
19. Restrepo-Garces CE, Marinov A, McHardy P, et al. Pulsed radiofrequency under ultrasound guidance for persistent stump-neuroma pain. Pain Pract 2011;11(1):98–102.
20. Nagaoka M, Matsuzaki H. Ultrasonography in tarsal tunnel syndrome. J Ultrasound Med 2005;24(8): 1035–40.
21. Girish G, Finlay K, Landry D, et al. Musculoskeletal disorders of the lower limb—ultrasound and magnetic resonance imaging correlation. Can Assoc Radiol J 2007;58(3):152–66.
22. Sofka CM, Collins AJ, Adler RS. Use of ultrasonographic guidance in interventional musculoskeletal procedures: a review from a single institution. J Ultrasound Med 2001;20(1):21–6.
23. Nagaoka M, Satou K. Tarsal tunnel syndrome caused by ganglia. J Bone Joint Surg Br 1999; 81(4):607–10.
24. Paavola M, Paakkala T, Kannus P, et al. Ultrasonography in the differential diagnosis of Achilles

tendon injuries and related disorders a comparison between pre-operative ultrasonography and surgical findings. Acta Radiol 1998;39(6):612–9.

25. Khan KM, Forster BB, Robinson J, et al. Are ultrasound and magnetic resonance imaging of value in assessment of Achilles tendon disorders? A two year prospective study. Br J Sports Med 2003; 37(2):149–53.

26. Taljanovic MS, Alcala JN, Gimber LH, et al. High-resolution US and MR imaging of peroneal tendon injuries. Radiographics 2015;35(1):179–99.

27. Amlang MH, Zwipp H, Friedrich A, et al. Ultrasonographic classification of Achilles tendon ruptures as a rationale for individual treatment selection. ISRN Orthop 2011;2011:869703.

28. Westin O, Nilsson Helander K, Grävare Silbernagel K, et al. Acute ultrasonography investigation to predict reruptures and outcomes in patients with an Achilles tendon rupture. Orthop J Sports Med 2016;4(10). 2325967116667920.

29. Lee SJ, Jacobson JA, Kim SM, et al. Ultrasound and MRI of the peroneal tendons and associated pathology. Skeletal Radiol 2013;42(9):1191–200.

30. Molini L, Bianchi S. US in peroneal tendon tear. J Ultrasound 2014;17(2):125–34.

31. Pesquer L, Guillo S, Poussange N, et al. Dynamic ultrasound of peroneal tendon instability. Br J Radiol 2016;89(1063):20150958.

32. Varghese A, Bianchi S. Ultrasound of tibialis anterior muscle and tendon: anatomy, technique of examination, normal and pathologic appearance. J Ultrasound 2014;17(2):113–23.

33. Lhoste-Trouilloud A. The tibialis posterior tendon. J Ultrasound 2012;15(1):2–6.

34. Gandjbakhch F, Terslev L, Joshua F, et al. Ultrasound in the evaluation of enthesitis: status and perspectives. Arthritis Res Ther 2011;13(6):R188.

35. Wiebking U, Pacha TO, Jagodzinski M. An accuracy evaluation of clinical, arthrometric, and stress-sonographic acute ankle instability examinations. Foot Ankle Surg 2015;21(1):42–8.

36. Maeda M, Maeda N, Takaoka T, et al. Sonographic findings of chondral avulsion fractures of the lateral ankle ligaments in children. J Ultrasound Med 2017; 36(2):421–32.

37. Reach JS, Easley ME, Chuckpaiwong B, et al. Accuracy of ultrasound guided injections in the foot and ankle. Foot Ankle Int 2009;30(3):239–42.

38. Wisniewski SJ, Smith J, Patterson DG, et al. Ultrasound-guided versus nonguided tibiotalar joint and sinus tarsi injections: a cadaveric study. PM R 2010;2(4):277–81.

39. Khosla S, Thiele R, Baumhauer JF. Ultrasound guidance for intra-articular injections of the foot and ankle. Foot Ankle Int 2009;30(9):886–90.

40. Gilliland CA, Salazar LD, Borchers JR. Ultrasound versus anatomic guidance for intra-articular and periarticular injection: a systematic review. Phys Sportsmed 2011;39(3):121–31.

41. Khoury NJ, el-Khoury GY, Saltzman CL, et al. Intra-articular foot and ankle injections to identify source of pain before arthrodesis. AJR Am J Roentgenol 1996;167(3):669–73.

42. Mitchell MJ, Bielecki D, Bergman AG, et al. Localization of specific joint causing hindfoot pain: value of injecting local anesthetics into individual joints during arthrography. AJR Am J Roentgenol 1995; 164(6):1473–6.

43. Stegeman M, van Ginneken BT, Boetes B, et al. Can diagnostic injections predict the outcome in foot and ankle arthrodesis? BMC Musculoskelet Disord 2014;15:11.

44. Ju BL, Weber KL, Khoury V. Ultrasound-guided therapy for knee and foot ganglion cysts. J Foot Ankle Surg 2017;56(1):153–7.

45. Saboeiro GR, Sofka CM. Ultrasound-guided ganglion cyst aspiration. HSS J 2008;4(2):161–3.

46. Kane D, Greaney T, Bresnihan B, et al. Ultrasound guided injection of recalcitrant plantar fasciitis. Ann Rheum Dis 1998;57(6):383–4.

47. Daftary AR, Karnik AS. Perspectives in ultrasound-guided musculoskeletal interventions. Indian J Radiol Imaging 2015;25(3):246–60.

48. Drakonaki EE, Allen GM, Watura R. Ultrasound-guided intervention in the ankle and foot. Br J Radiol 2016;89(1057):20150577.

49. Vallone G, Vittorio T. Complete Achilles tendon rupture after local infiltration of corticosteroids in the treatment of deep retrocalcaneal bursitis. J Ultrasound 2014;17(2):165–7.

50. Maxwell NJ, Ryan MB, Taunton JE, et al. Sonographically guided intratendinous injection of hyperosmolar dextrose to treat chronic tendinosis of the Achilles tendon: a pilot study. AJR Am J Roentgenol 2007;189(4):W215–20.

51. Guevara-Alvarez A, Schmitt A, Russell RP, et al. Growth factor delivery vehicles for tendon injuries: mesenchymal stem cells and platelet rich plasma. Muscles Ligaments Tendons J 2014;4(3): 378–85.

52. Wu PT, Lee JS, Wu KC, et al. Ultrasound-guided percutaneous radiofrequency lesioning when treating recalcitrant plantar fasciitis: clinical results. Ultraschall Med 2016;37(1):56–62.

53. Isner-Horobeti ME, Dufour SP, Blaes C, et al. Intramuscular pressure before and after botulinum toxin in chronic exertional compartment syndrome of the leg: a preliminary study. Am J Sports Med 2013; 41(11):2558–66.

54. Huang YC, Wei SH, Wang HK, et al. Ultrasonographic guided botulinum toxin type A treatment for plantar fasciitis: an outcome-based investigation for treating pain and gait changes. J Rehabil Med 2010;42(2):136–40.

55. Finnoff JT, Rajasekaran S. Ultrasound-guided, percutaneous needle fascial fenestration for the treatment of chronic exertional compartment syndrome: a case report. PM R 2016;8(3):286–90.

56. Morgan PA, Monaghan GA, Richards S. A systematic review of ultrasound-guided and non ultrasound-guided therapeutic injections to treat Morton's neuroma. J Am Podiatr Med Assoc 2014;104(4):337–48.

57. Chuter GS, Chua YP, Connell DA, et al. Ultrasound-guided radiofrequency ablation in the management of interdigital (Morton's) neuroma. Skeletal Radiol 2013;42(1):107–11.

58. Mortada MA, Solyman A, Elsayed SB. SAT0404 efficacy and safety of hydrodissection of median nerve as a treatment of idiopathic carpal tunnel syndrome. Ann Rheum Dis 2013;72:A719–20.

59. Makhlouf T, Emil NS, Sibbitt WL Jr, et al. Outcomes and cost-effectiveness of carpal tunnel injections using sonographic needle guidance. Clin Rheumatol 2014;33(6):849–58.

60. Fader RR, Mitchell JJ, Chadayammuri VP, et al. Percutaneous ultrasound-guided hydrodissection of a symptomatic sural neuroma. Orthopedics 2015;38(11):e1046–50.

61. Park HJ, Lee SM, Lee SY, et al. Ultrasound-guided percutaneous removal of wooden foreign bodies in the extremities with hydro-dissection technique. Korean J Radiol 2015;16(6):1326–31.

62. Leung A, Patton A, Navoy J, et al. Intraoperative sonography-guided removal of radiolucent foreign bodies. J Pediatr Orthop 1998;18(2):259–61.

63. Budhram GR, Schmunk JC. Bedside ultrasound AIDS identification and removal of cutaneous foreign bodies: a case series. J Emerg Med 2014; 47(2):e43–8.

64. Paziana K, Fields JM, Rotte M, et al. Soft tissue foreign body removal technique using portable ultrasonography. Wilderness Environ Med 2012;23(4): 343–8.

65. Chan O, O'Dowd D, Padhiar N, et al. High volume image guided injections in chronic Achilles tendinopathy. Disabil Rehabil 2008;30(20–22): 1697–708.

66. Maffulli N, Spiezia F, Longo UG, et al. High volume image guided injections for the management of chronic tendinopathy of the main body of the Achilles tendon. Phys Ther Sport 2013; 14(3):163–7.

67. Alfredson H. Low recurrence rate after mini surgery outside the tendon combined with short rehabilitation in patients with midportion Achilles tendinopathy. Open Access J Sports Med 2016;7:51–4.

68. Paczesny ŁM, Kruczyński J. Ultrasound-guided arthroscopic management of hallux rigidus. Wideochir Inne Tech Maloinwazyjne 2016;11(3):144–8.

69. Vohra PK, Japour CJ. Ultrasound-guided plantar fascia release technique: a retrospective study of 46 feet. J Am Podiatr Med Assoc 2009;99(3):183–90.

70. Ohuchi H, Ichikawa K, Shinga K, et al. Ultrasound-assisted endoscopic partial plantar fascia release. Arthrosc Tech 2013;2(3):e227–30.

71. Patel MM. A novel treatment for refractory plantar fasciitis. Am J Orthop (Belle Mead NJ) 2015;44(3): 107–10.

72. Pourcho AM, Hall MM. Percutaneous ultrasonic fasciotomy for refractory plantar fasciopathy after failure of a partial endoscopic release procedure. PM R 2015;7(11):1194–7.

73. Chou AC, Ng SY, Su DH, et al. Radiofrequency microtenotomy is as effective as plantar fasciotomy in the treatment of recalcitrant plantar fasciitis. Foot Ankle Surg 2016;22(4):270–3.

74. Lucas DE, Ekroth SR, Hyer CF. Intermediate-term results of partial plantar fascia release with microtenotomy using bipolar radiofrequency microtenotomy. J Foot Ankle Surg 2015;54(2):179–82.

75. Sorensen MD, Hyer CF, Philbin TM. Percutaneous bipolar radiofrequency microdebridement for recalcitrant proximal plantar fasciosis. J Foot Ankle Surg 2011;50(2):165–70.

76. Erken HY, Ayanoglu S, Akmaz I, et al. Prospective study of percutaneous radiofrequency nerve ablation for chronic plantar fasciitis. Foot Ankle Int 2014;35(2):95–103.

77. Hormozi J, Lee S, Hong DK. Minimal invasive percutaneous bipolar radiofrequency for plantar fasciotomy: a retrospective study. J Foot Ankle Surg 2011;50(3):283–6.

78. Villanueva M, Iborra Á, Rodríguez G, et al. Ultrasound-guided gastrocnemius recession: a new ultra-minimally invasive surgical technique. BMC Musculoskelet Disord 2016;17(1):409.

79. Lueders DR, Sellon JL, Smith J, et al. Ultrasound-guided fasciotomy for chronic exertional compartment syndrome: a cadaveric investigation. PM R 2017;9(7):683–90.

80. Gousse RP, Beard NM, Hyden JC. Right percutaneous fasciotomy and osteotomy for plantar fasciosis and enthesophyte fracture nonunion. Poster presented at: National Conference of the American Medical Society of Sports Medicine. San Diego, May 8–13, 2017.

81. Pilecki Z, Koczy B, Mielnik M, et al. Basic dissecting techniques in ultrasound-guided surgery. J Ultrason 2014;14(57):171–8.

Moving?

Make sure your subscription moves with you!

To notify us of your new address, find your **Clinics Account Number** (located on your mailing label above your name), and contact customer service at:

Email: journalscustomerservice-usa@elsevier.com

800-654-2452 (subscribers in the U.S. & Canada)
314-447-8871 (subscribers outside of the U.S. & Canada)

Fax number: 314-447-8029

Elsevier Health Sciences Division
Subscription Customer Service
3251 Riverport Lane
Maryland Heights, MO 63043

ELSEVIER

Printed and bound by CPI Group (UK) Ltd, Croydon, CR0 4YY

08/05/2025

01864703-0017

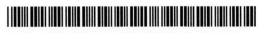